Praise for IFS Health Therapy

"For those living with chronic illness who ever wondered whether they possessed any real agency over the course of their condition, this book is for you. Written by three experts in their fields, it guides the reader through a well-researched and explained path toward healing. This is an essential addition to any thoughtful bookshelf."

—**Nancy A. Shadick, MD, MPH,** Division of Rheumatology, Inflammation & Immunity, Brigham & Women's Hospital; associate professor of medicine, Harvard Medical School

"As the first book describing the intersection of IFS therapy and health and illness, this is a must-read for clinicians but also serves as a compassionate and hopeful companion for those suffering with pain and chronic illnesses. Nancy Sowell picks up the thread from her collaboration in the groundbreaking IFS research study demonstrating improved outcomes for patients with rheumatoid arthritis. Readers are walked thoroughly through the compassionate process of IFS health therapy to show us how well-being is possible for those with chronic illness."

—**Cece Sykes, LCSW,** primary author of *IFS Therapy for Addictions* and senior IFS trainer

"Scientific research increasingly demonstrates that early life trauma and stress contribute to the onset and perpetuation of chronic illness. In *IFS Health Therapy*, the authors bring decades of combined experience working with clients using the innovative IFS model to alleviate the impacts of trauma and stress among people with chronic health conditions. Nancy Sowell led the experimental intervention for the first randomized controlled trial of IFS at Brigham and Women's Hospital, which was published in 2013. The study demonstrated reductions in depression and improved quality of life among people with rheumatoid arthritis. Since that time, those of us who treat and research how to support people living with chronic illness have eagerly awaited this book's publication. Learning how to calmly be with symptoms of chronic illness, how to have compassion for parts reacting to living with the illness, and how to alleviate the toxic stress affecting the mind and body are at the core of not just surviving but thriving. This book lays out a compelling relationally driven approach to help readers learn how to do that themselves."

—**Zev Schuman-Olivier, MD,** founding director of the Center for Mindfulness and Compassion, medical director of outpatient addictions, and director of addiction research at Cambridge Health Alliance; associate professor in psychiatry at Harvard Medical School

"Nancy Sowell has written a groundbreaking and humane guide to understanding the indelible relationship between physical and psychological healing. Meticulously researched and lucidly written, this book should be required reading for anyone who suffers from chronic illness, pain, or the symptoms of unhealed trauma. That is, it should be required reading for almost everyone, but especially those interested in taking an active role in their own recovery. Destined to become a modern classic of health literature, it has already become a precious touchstone for me."

—**Melissa Febos,** author of *The Dry Season* and *Girlhood*, winner of the National Book Critics Circle Award, and Roy J. Carver professor and director of the Nonfiction Writing Program at the University of Iowa

"This book is a thoughtful and important extension of IFS into the realm of physical health and illness. Nancy Sowell, along with her coauthors, brings a grounded, respectful voice to this work. She writes with clarity and compassion, honoring the protective roles of parts and the innate wisdom within every system. The book offers clinicians and clients a gentle yet impactful way to listen and restore internal balance to parts injured by trauma and other burdens that dysregulate the body and affect health."

—Toni Herbine-Blank, MSN, developer of Intimacy from the Inside Out (IFS-based relationship therapy) and coauthor of the *IFS Couple Therapy Skills Manual*

"Nancy Sowell has been one of the most important teachers of my career. The tools she has taught me have transformed my practice and the lives of my patients. Now, in this book, she has made those tools available to everyone. Written with Martha Sweezy and Richard Schwartz, it does what I have searched for across decades of practice: it explains, clearly and scientifically and with deep compassion, why our patients suffer the way they do—and what can actually help. Grounded in solid science and rare clinical wisdom, it traces the path from early adversity through the nervous system to the symptoms that fill our offices, and back out again through IFS-informed tools that work. The people who encounter these techniques will find not just symptom relief, but a fundamentally different relationship with their own suffering. This is a gift to every healer and to every person who seeks their help. I am deeply grateful to these authors for writing it."

—Charles Silberstein, MD, medical director, Martha's Vineyard Community Services; Martha's Vineyard Hospital, Department of Psychiatry

"*IFS Health Therapy* is a clear, compassionate, and deeply practical guide to understanding the mind–body system through the lens of IFS. The authors illuminate how trauma, chronic stress, and shame shape internal experience, offering a nuanced explanation of autonomic states, chronic arousal, and allostatic overload. Although written for a broad audience, its insights into chronic stress pathways have powerful implications for understanding the cumulative impact of racial trauma on communities of the global majority. Readers and clinicians working with members of the global majority will find the framework especially helpful for recognizing how protectors adapt to ongoing experiences of discrimination, systemic inequities, and intergenerational stress—and how, through the healing of exiled parts, these burdens can be witnessed, unburdened, and transformed. *IFS Health Therapy* stands out as a comprehensive, invaluable, and highly relevant resource for clinicians and anyone interested in healing through IFS."

—Tamala Floyd, LCSW, IFS psychotherapist and author of *Listening When Parts Speak: A Practical Guide to Healing with Internal Family Systems Therapy and Ancestor Wisdom*

"*IFS Health Therapy* offers a much-needed map for clinicians entering the complex terrain of chronic stress and illness. Its nuanced case studies will be of considerable value to both experienced clinicians and those new to the model. My physician parts relax in the presence of this depathologizing and compassionate approach and feel hope toward shifting the language of 'difficult to treat' to 'What's going on here?' The authors beautifully weave scientific knowledge with their extensive clinical wisdom in a gift to us all."

—Risa Adams, MD, IFSI trainer and coauthor of *It Doesn't Have to Be This Way: A Physician's Guide to Radical Self Care*

"My experience as a national women's rugby player who has had multiple injuries and my 30 years as a muscular therapist have shown me that injury and chronic pain are rarely just physical. Pain has a story that's often accompanied by emotional trauma. This book provides the language for understanding that experience. The IFS-based treatment shows the reader how 'parts' live not only in the mind, but in the body, and how their healing can bring physical as well as emotional relief. I'm especially inspired by the potential for interdisciplinary collaboration. When IFS-informed psychotherapists and bodyworkers begin to share a common map, the possibility for client care expands in powerful ways. This book feels like an important step toward that future—one where healing is truly integrated across disciplines."

—Mary Gail Sullivan, former captain of the US women's national rugby team (Rugby World Cup winners, 1991); muscular therapist and former instructor at the Muscular Therapy Institute of Cambridge, MA

IFS [Internal Family Systems] Health Therapy

Treating Trauma-Related Physical Illness & Toxic Stress

Nancy Sowell, LICSW, with
Martha Sweezy, PhD, & Richard C. Schwartz, PhD

IFS (INTERNAL FAMILY SYSTEMS) HEALTH THERAPY

Published by
PESI Publishing, Inc.
3839 White Ave
Eau Claire, WI 54703

Cover and interior design by Emily Dyer
Editing by Jenessa Jackson, PhD

ISBN 9781683739333 (print)
ISBN 9781683739340 (ePUB)
ISBN 9781683739357 (ePDF)

Printed in the United States of America.

PESI Publishing
pesipublishing.com

To those who suffer with chronic health conditions related to the toxic stress of unmet developmental needs from neglect or any form of trauma, growing up under harsh circumstances, or with too much pressure, fear, or shaming messages—this book is dedicated to you.

—Nancy Sowell

I dedicate my efforts in this book to my friends Steffie Woolhandler, MD, and David Himmelstein, MD, who founded Physicians for a National Health Program (PNHP), spearheading the movement for single-payer health care in the United States, and have dedicated their careers to making good medical care available to all.

—Martha Sweezy

I dedicate this book to my late father, Ted Schwartz, MD, who piqued my interest in applying IFS to medical conditions and who guided me throughout the journey.

—Richard C. Schwartz

Table of Contents

Preface

—Richard C. Schwartz, PhD—

When I developed Internal Family Systems (IFS) therapy, I focused on the inner conflicts of self-critical, despairing people. I did not set out to create a model for physical healing. Yet over the years, this huge topic refused to stay at the margins of my work. As people accessed their Self, and their parts unburdened, their bodies often changed even though this was never an explicit goal of therapy. Chronic pain softened. Autoimmune flares quieted. Sleep improved. Energy returned. My clients were thrilled with these seeming side effects of the IFS process, and I was also gratified. My family is highly medical. My father was a physician, as are three of my brothers. As the eldest of the brothers, I was supposed to have a medical career, but I didn't have the grades for medical school or an inclination for medicine. My self-esteem and my family's respect were both elevated by the discovery that IFS can ameliorate some medical symptoms.

Although the phenomenon was not universal and the physical shifts that did occur were not predictable, they happened often and consistently enough. I had to admit something important was happening at the interface between psyche and soma. I was not alone in this. Among others, Nancy Sowell homed in, integrated IFS with her behavioral medicine training, spearheaded the first IFS health study, and produced this book. I'm so grateful to Nancy for her continued commitment to using IFS for physical healing and for her expertise in this area.

Rather than asking whether chronic illness is "psychological" or "medical," this book starts from the premise that our systems are fully integrated at all levels of being. We who practice IFS now know that long-standing patterns of stress, including from burdensome beliefs and extreme protector behaviors, influence the body in profound ways. Vigilant, suppressive, terrified, sad, and enraged parts can activate the nervous system for decades on end. When feelings are invalidated and memories exiled, the body pays the price. Burdens have radical effects within the body. Vulnerable parts who are frozen in trauma scenes and trembling with terror will affect your body no matter how hard your protectors work to forget, eat well, exercise, or meditate.

In addition, once all your parts feel seen and heard by you and have been retrieved from the past, they won't need to use physical vulnerabilities to get your attention or protect other parts. It's equally true that IFS can't and won't improve every condition. For example, many of us have genetic predispositions or catch viruses that manifest as illness regardless of how we treat our parts. But even then, we can help protective parts who might react to such a challenge in some inadvertently injurious way.

Crucially, IFS is not about eliminating parts, their feelings, or their protective adaptations. Rather, it brings immense resources to a depleted inner system and shifts internal relationships. When protectors are able to calm down, exiles can be witnessed and validated and the Self can become a consistent inner leader.

Self-leadership—which means the mind is no longer a stress-inducing battleground for polarized parts—helps free the body to recover.

This book does not make grand promises. IFS will not replace medical care. We who practice IFS value inquiry into both lived experience and science. We have seen IFS reduce chronic stress, enhance interoceptive awareness, and restore the sense of internal safety in people who are suffering long-term health conditions. In the service of healing, we aim for the Self of client and therapist to partner with health professionals from all disciplines.

Equally important, we are concerned with the dignity of people who have chronic illnesses. Most of us have been blamed, subtly or otherwise, for experiencing symptoms. Sometimes we've been told, explicitly or implicitly, that we would be well if we were less stressed, more positive, or more disciplined. In IFS the message is different. Symptomatic behaviors guide us to motives, which reveal the underlying problem and open the door to solutions. Although parts are often unaware of their somatic impact and people are often unaware of their parts, symptoms always make sense in the context where they developed, which will include an internal system doing its best to survive. Truly received, this message resolves shame and invites healing.

So, here's our invitation. Let's see the mind and body as they truly are: interactive, integrated, and adaptive. If you are in the business of promoting health—perhaps as a psychotherapist, a psychiatrist, a medical doctor, or some other profession related to disease prevention—and you'd like a new perspective on emotional stress and physiology that involves maximal internal resources, read this book. You may encounter some welcome surprises—we sure have.

Introduction

Early adversity in the form of chronic stress or trauma has been linked to persistent systemic inflammation in the body and many common diseases. These include cardiac disease and cancer as well as autoimmune diseases, diabetes, and more. In this book, we use the words *stress* and *trauma* to refer to a broad range of experiences, including various forms of neglect (e.g., lack of attention, emotional holding, or adult guidance) as well as physical, sexual, and emotional abuse. We also use these terms to refer to the categorical insults that many of us experience, such as racism, homophobia, and misogyny, as well as more material trauma that can affect individuals and communities, such as the economic and political cataclysm of war or the life-threatening effects of climate change.

Like so many of our clients, adverse experiences in childhood contributed to our health difficulties both early and later in life. For example, one of the authors of this book, Nancy, grew up in a household with financial insecurity and lack of resources. Coping with income inequality and long work hours, her single mother left her alone to navigate various challenges and dangers, such as bullying and abusive caretakers. She developed psoriasis and, later on, psoriatic arthritis, a disabling autoimmune disease. She remembers the increasing pain, the struggle to walk, and the frustration of a misdiagnosis, but what stands out most is the fear. This health challenge sparked a reckoning for her as an adult: "How did I get here? Why is this happening? What do I do now?"

Coping with physical pain, fear, and the grinding process of getting an accurate diagnosis, Nancy used Internal Family Systems (IFS) therapy to address underlying trauma-related issues. Her coauthor, Richard Schwartz, has done the same. Schwartz created IFS, which is a nonpathologizing model of psychotherapy that guides therapists and clients to find and help wounded parts (a.k.a. subpersonalities) within. The wounds come from the stress overload that grows when developmental needs like nurturance, support, and safety go unmet, and when children are subjected to physical, sexual, and emotional transgressions. As we illustrate, these stressors can contribute a lot to physical disease.

Difficult circumstances and painful experiences lead parts within the internal family system to take on protective roles to shield us from further harm. Despite the parts' good intentions, the messages and behaviors they turn to can foster the feared outcome. For example, someone who is repeatedly criticized by their caretakers might develop a part that strives relentlessly for success. While this hard-driving part is trying to counter the underlying fear of failure, it will likely end up overwhelming the system and causing burnout. We find that protective parts like that striver are generally willing to relax if we forgo directing and judging them in favor of listening to them with interest. When we are consistent about receiving and learning nonjudgmentally from our internal system, our parts will usually (if cautiously) let go of painful, distorted beliefs about their self-worth, safety, and potential. This allows the *mind-body* (the term we use to capture the complex intertwining of mind and body) to compose and heal, opening the way for better physical and mental health.

In this book, readers will find case illustrations, in-depth commentary, experiential exercises, and clinical tools that illustrate how IFS therapy can be used to address unmet developmental needs, attachment wounds, and trauma that can result in physical illness and health problems. Known as *IFS health therapy*, it is intended for healthcare providers of all disciplines as well as anyone interested in the application of IFS to improve health. Clients, too, can use the experiential exercises to deepen their internal awareness, recognize and find different subpersonality parts, and access their inherent wisdom and capacity to heal.

This book is divided into seven chapters, beginning with explanations of core concepts and progressing through guidance for each phase of IFS health therapy:

- **Chapter 1** covers the foundational principles of IFS therapy by introducing the difference between various parts (managers, fighters, exiles) and the Self and discussing how to communicate with parts. It also provides an initial introduction to the healing protocol behind the IFS health therapy approach that we use in this book.

- **Chapter 2** describes how trauma, chronic stress, and shame get under our skin and affect the parts of the internal system. We describe the role of different autonomic nervous system states and the link between chronic autonomic arousal and allostatic overload.

- **Chapter 3** offers step-by-step guidance on how to conduct an IFS health therapy assessment with a distressed internal system, introduce clients to the IFS health therapy approach, set initial goals, and interface with other health professionals and systems.

- **Chapter 4** describes IFS health therapy as a relational healing process and emphasizes the importance of establishing the therapeutic relationship to set the stage for treatment. It also discusses how to use the chronic stress cycle to familiarize yourself with parts who are most relevant to the client's illness.

- **Chapter 5** introduces the first phase of IFS health therapy—working with protectors—and is chock full of case illustrations, theoretical explanations, and descriptions of techniques to help you identify and befriend the protective parts who influence health.

- **Chapter 6** moves on to the second phase of IFS health therapy: healing the wounded exiles through the unburdening process. Here, we walk you through the first five steps of unburdening (witnessing, rescripting, retrieval, unburdening ritual, invitation) through a series of case illustrations.

- **Chapter 7** concludes with the third and final phase of IFS health therapy—integration—which represents the last step of the unburdening process. This phase shifts the developmental journey from chronic stress and illness to a life of enriching pursuits and nourishing relationships, inside and out.

Throughout these chapters, we provide case stories illustrating the IFS health treatment course—from the beginning of therapy to its final stages—with clients with different health problems, including metabolic syndrome, autoimmune diseases, and chronic pain and somatic symptom–related health problems. These cases show how to heal from a painful past, unburden parts and the body, and create a life in balance to support health and well-being.

We conceived this book in a spirit of respect and appreciation for medical science, aiming to illustrate how adversity alters a person's mind and body, affecting their physical health. Clients who are suffering physically as well as emotionally have many challenges. Nonetheless, we propose hope. Trauma does not damage the Self, which is the goodness and healing capacity within each of us. The Self heals and revives parts. Their release, in turn, frees the body to regain its natural balance and vitality. We invite you to join us and learn more about this approach to physical health.

[CHAPTER 1]

Core IFS Concepts

The IFS Model of Mind Is Plural

Therapists who practice IFS see the mind as naturally divided. Since clients speak of their *parts*, we follow suit. We understand parts as mental entities with fully formed personalities that come online developmentally throughout life—in everyone. In some ways, parts are like people. Each of them has its own traits, temperament, interests, preferences, gifts, and vulnerabilities. They live in a social web, fulfilling socially determined roles in their system, allying with each other, and getting into conflict (best known to mental health practitioners as *intrapsychic conflict*). They live largely behind a veil, out of awareness, but external events and social systems affect them, and they are fully capable of forming deep interpersonal bonds and communicating interpersonally.

Of course, in other ways, parts are not like people. They can influence the material world, but they are not of it. They can shape-shift, appear and disappear from consciousness, use any of the senses to communicate, and, unless they're stuck at some point in the past, travel through time freely. Relative to our hobbled capacities on the material plane, they are magicians of time and space. If you wish to find and connect with a part, try noticing it when it comes forward. How are you aware of its presence? Perhaps it shows up as an action urge, a mood, a perception, a thought, or a sensation. All of these signal a part's existence.

There are many other ways to find parts too. You might notice when one part recedes and another takes over, causing your mood or thoughts to change. You might notice contradictory thoughts or behaviors that signify a heated disagreement between parts. You might favor one feature of your personality or behavior (one part) over another because you're seeing through the eyes of a part who believes strongly in its perspective. Conversely, you might dislike or disapprove of some behavior or feature of your personality, which means you're seeing that part through the eyes of another who is critical. Regardless of how your parts appear and behave, all of them have positive intentions for you. They are dedicated to you and to their internal community. They do what they can to keep you functioning, external forces notwithstanding. They are, as Schwartz says, sacred inner beings.

Parts and Their Jobs

Managers

Starting from infancy, when one part gets hurt, other parts assume the job of trying to ensure the internal system's safety. These proactive protectors, which we call *managers* because they organize and direct our lives, are principally invested in relationships, appearances, and social standing. They work to constrain and control the strong feelings or socially challenging behavior of other parts. If a vulnerable part believes it is unlovable and worthless as a result of being devalued, managers don't have the capacity or authority to challenge and counteract that outcome (they're as likely to believe these insults as the injured part), so they work hard to banish this part and its suffering from consciousness. Accordingly, we call these wounded, vulnerable parts *exiles*, which we'll talk more about in a bit.

Managers may not have the wherewithal to heal exiles, but they do try to prevent future wounding in various ways, including with insistent warnings about danger and efforts to improve or hide exiles. Often, they rely on shaming tactics (Sweezy, 2023). They can also ramp up anxiety on purpose, promote avoidance behaviors, smother with silencing concern, banish knowledge (what Freud called *repression*), interrupt thoughts and feelings with dissociative fog, tweak the body to produce physical symptoms, and do many other consequential things. However, their most reliable go-to tactics are criticism, judgment, and warnings that external others are doing the judging. Managers are not all harsh and extreme in these ways—many are benign helpers in everyday life—but harsh inhibitions are the norm for protective managers who fear danger. Their inhibitions generate another set of problems, as they instigate a different type of protector to emerge in response: firefighters.

Qualities of Managers

- Keenly observe what works in different social environments (e.g., home, school)
- Worry about consequences
- Observe and copy the behaviors of authority figures
- Adjust their behavior to the external environment
- Rely on inhibition and shaming inside and out (e.g., warnings, criticism, control, denial)
- Suppress the unmet needs of vulnerable parts
- Plan and set a course of action to maintain control
- Work hard to banish troublesome parts, both exiles and reactive firefighters

Firefighters

To counterbalance the negative effects of excessive inhibition while keeping exiled pain out of mind, another set of protectors emerges. We call these reactive protectors *firefighters* because they'll knock down the house to put out the fire—rebelling with various distracting disinhibitions that are effective in the short run but exact great costs from relationships and the body over time. These include blaming and raging against others, taking sexual or other risks, self-harming, and soothing or numbing with addictive processes like over- or undereating, substance use, pornography, or gambling. Essentially, when the fear-mongering, rule-setting, and *shoulds* of managers become too encompassing and oppressive, firefighters rebelliously champion *wants*.

Their decisions and behaviors offer momentary satisfaction and immediate relief but can exact a social, physical, or psychological toll that directly or secondarily affects the internal social system and health. They typically win the battle for immediate relief but lose the war on shame and vulnerability because banishing burdened exiles and prolonging internal conflicts with managers prevents the system from achieving relational, emotional, and physiological resolution of trauma and unmet needs. Firefighters' tendency to utilize substances and extreme behavior to soothe fear, loneliness, and longing can lead to more mental and physical vulnerability.

Some firefighters who had to deal with external abusers absorbed some of that energy in order to survive the harsh environment. Their protective strategies can mirror that of the original perpetrator, creating an internally stressed environment that is hard on relationships, other parts, and the body. Firefighter strategies like aggression or suicidality can be highly triggering, while others are socially acceptable and even promoted, like overworking, overusing screens, dieting, and exercising. However, even these supposedly good habits will be destructive to our health and well-being when used excessively to quell erupting vulnerability. Firefighters will use whatever works to gain control, including the symptoms of an illness.

Qualities of Firefighters

- Counterbalance managerial inhibition with disinhibition
- Attend to wants and desires
- Push for relaxation and fun
- Escalate to match the extremism of managers
- Dissociate and distract when exiled pain surfaces
- Soothe by overusing and overconsuming (e.g., food, drugs, screens, porn, exercise, sex, rage)
- Absorb the harsh negative energy of abusers to protect other parts
- Care only for immediate relief

Exiles

As we've discussed, exiles are the vulnerable parts of the system. They are usually burdened by negative feelings and beliefs about their value and stuck in the past. Exiles are in pain and full of longing. They have suffered from some traumatic loss or shaming insult (e.g., neglect, physical violence, sexual assault). Their needs for attention, validation, love, support, and connection have been unmet. They feel unlovable.

Since managers and firefighters use different tactics, they're often mutually disapproving and their conflicts can escalate to alarming heights. They both aim to deliver us from pain, but because their project never fully succeeds, they can't ever stop. An exile clamors for recognition and care. In response, managers double down on shaming, which inflames the exile's sense of shamefulness and inspires firefighters to soothe and distract as needed. The cycle continues with managers ramping up again to shame the shameless firefighters, and on it goes (Sweezy, 2023). Over time, this exhausting cycle grows ever more habitual and hair trigger, leaving people hard-pressed to slow down and inspect their mental processes at arm's length on their own. When we're in it, we often need outside help to get out, which is why therapists continue to have clients.

Shame Cycle

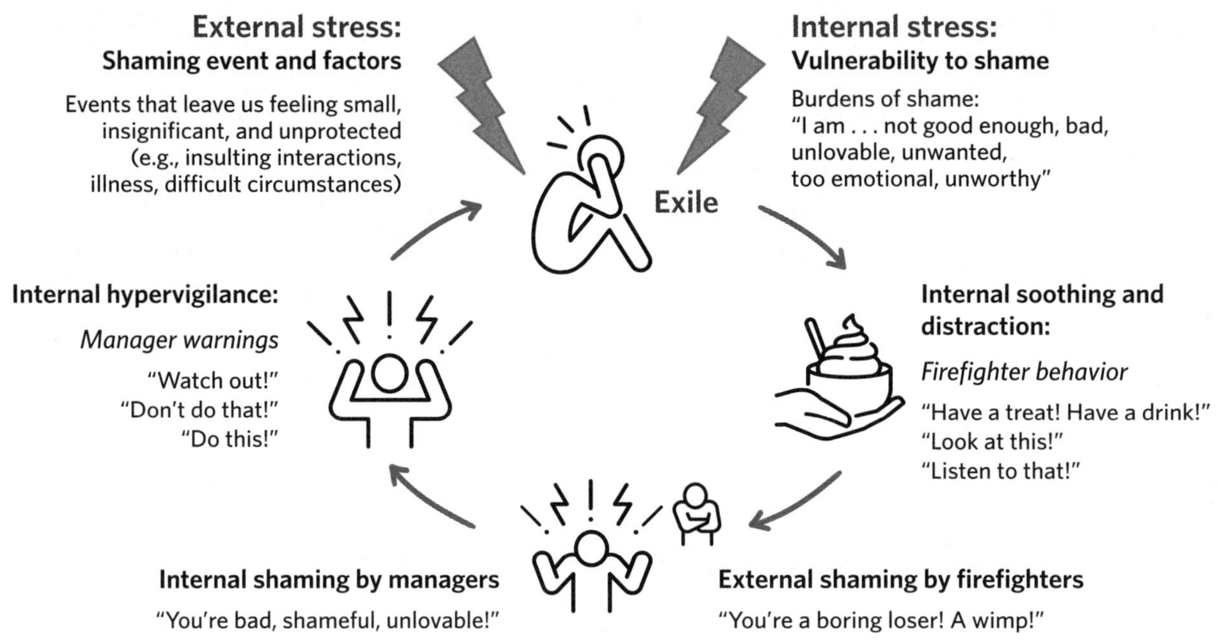

When we grow up with safe relationships and adequate resources, our parts are not pushed to these extremes. We're able to relax, explore, and keep learning, which is the foundation for lifelong physical and mental health. However, when resources are scarce, stress is chronic, and fear is foremost, parts don't fare so well. They feel alone, disposable, and ashamed. Managers fear this state of mind above all. They don't want wounded, despairing parts causing a collapse, and they don't want a firefighter lashing out in counteractive rage. Yet though they have the power to banish hurt parts from awareness, sometimes for decades, they can't prevent the profound effect those parts have on the psyche and interdependent biological systems. Exiles are the linchpin of suffering. Once they feel better, protectors can relax and the body can heal. But who can help an exile? Luckily for us, there is more to the mind than parts.

Self

When parts relax their grip on the body and mind, we slide into a different state of consciousness characterized by awareness and acceptance. In this state, we feel centered and calm, and we are curious or compassionate rather than judgmental toward our parts and other people. Since clients often speak of this manifestation of consciousness as "my core self" or "the real me," we call it the *Self*, with a capital S to designate its unique nature and differentiate it from other uses of the word.* The Self is characterized by open-minded, nonjudgmental qualities like kindness and what Schwartz dubbed the *8 C's* (curiosity, confidence, courage, connectedness, creativity, calm, clarity, and compassion), as well as the *5 P's* (patience, presence, playfulness, perspective, and persistence). The Self's inner leadership restores internal balance and peace, soothes biological systems, and helps the internal system respond with equanimity to the ups and downs of relationships and chance.

IFS aims for the client's Self to connect with exiled parts and meet their needs. Protectors will allow this when they feel connected and safe, but to get connected, they must be willing to *unblend* or separate and be in relationship with the Self. We persuade them to unblend by being nonjudgmental, listening to their experiences, asking about their motives, and validating their good intentions.

Self: Unblends Protectors, Unburdens Exiles, and Brings Balance to the Mind-Body

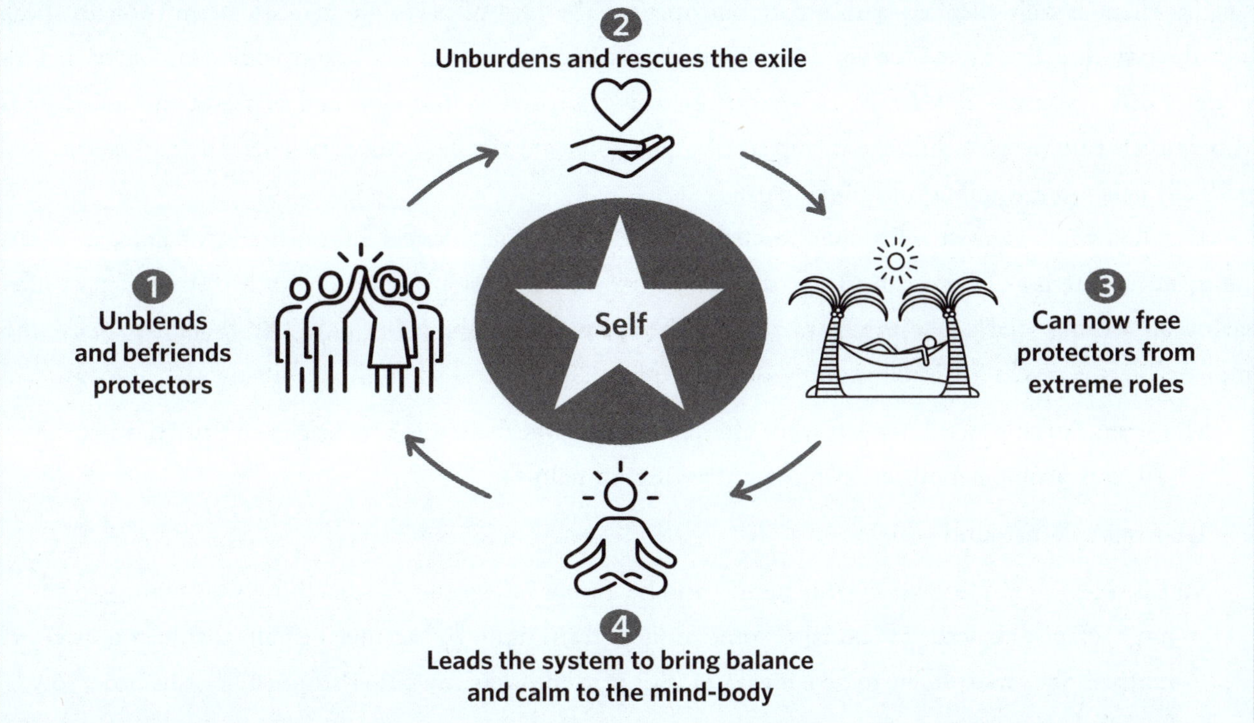

Communicating with Parts

IFS teaches two different ways of communicating with parts: *insight* and *direct access*. Insight is only possible if parts are willing to unblend. When they are willing, the Self shows up and is available. Once a client can embody their Self, we guide them to attend inward and find a part—in a physical sensation, thought, feeling, or behavior—they'd like to interview. The client with enough access to their Self will be patient,

* One client described the Self this way: "In my Self, I feel calm inside yet energized. I'm wide awake, but not in a vigilant way. It's peaceful. My heart feels open . . . The tension in my shoulders relaxes. I can breathe."

curious, and, eventually, compassionate. As an experience, insight can be intuitive and telepathic, sensory, auditory, or visual. Our motto is: Whatever works.

While it's natural for parts to blend, it's also natural for them to move in and out of our awareness. If a part won't unblend, we won't be aware of it—we will speak and act from the part. When this happens in therapy, the therapist can speak to the part directly, using the third person to talk about the client. We call this *direct access*, and we use it as a bridge to insight. When a client's protectors don't trust anyone, they may need this direct relationship with the therapist's Self for quite some time. It's a good way for the therapist to build credibility.

Direct access comes in two modes. The first is *implicit*. When a client is fully blended with a part and the part doesn't want to talk about parts, the therapist can talk with the blended part as if it is the client (e.g., "You seem frustrated. What's happening?"). This sounds like regular talk therapy. The difference is in the therapist, who speaks from their Self and views this as a conversation with just one of many parts. Implicit direct access is used at the very start of therapy and can occur at the beginning of a session as a transition from the day's activities into therapy.

If a client is fully blended with a part but open to the idea of parts, we can ask permission to speak with the part directly (e.g., "I see you have a frustrated part. How about I talk to it while you listen?"). This mode of direct access is called *explicit*. We can use this approach to interview and befriend embodied parts who won't yet unblend. While the therapist asks questions and the part talks, the client listens, learns, and gradually gets more separation from the part.

The following vignette illustrates implicit and explicit direct access in practice. Melanie, a white, transgender, heterosexual woman in her thirties, arrives at the session blended with a distressed part after having an asthma attack. She begins to tell the therapist a story about her day. The therapist sticks with implicit direct access at first, transitioning later to explicit direct access when she intuits the part is ready.

Melanie: I'm so upset! I just left work after a long day and there was a message from my brother, Gil, complaining about my parents and asking for help.

Therapist: What kind of help?

Melanie: Money. He always wants money and he always has a reason. Something went wrong, it's not his fault, he needs to "borrow" some money. Yeah, right! I guarantee he's already been to my mother. She's most likely to give it to him. But it sounds like my father stopped her this time, so he called me.

Therapist: What do you feel?

Melanie: Angry!

Therapist: You haven't talked much about anger. I'm glad you're sharing this today.

Melanie: This routine with my brother and mother—it really pisses me off!

Therapist: I hear that. And you've been dealing with it for a long time.

Melanie: Yes.

THERAPIST: This angry part hasn't gotten much attention from us yet.

Starting to use the word part while acknowledging and validating the part

MELANIE: No, it hasn't. And the situation hasn't changed! [*Her voice gets louder.*] I've *had it* with my mother enabling Gil!

THERAPIST: Would the angry part like some attention from you today?

Inviting the part to unblend

MELANIE: [*Turns her attention inward and pauses.*] I'm feeling it. It's too intense to back down.

An indication that other parts are pushing back against the angry part

THERAPIST: How about I talk with this angry part directly and you listen? [*Melanie nods.*] Just let the part be you.

Asking permission before switching to explicit direct access

MELANIE: [*Closes her eyes, pauses.*] Okay.

THERAPIST: You're the part of Melanie who's had it with Gil and her mother. [*She nods.*] What do you want us to understand?

MELANIE'S ANGRY PART: This is never going to change. No one stands up to Gil. Everyone treats him like a 16-year-old and enables his drinking. He's a man in his 30s!

THERAPIST: Have you wanted to stand up to him?

MELANIE'S ANGRY PART: For years! I can't stand the way my parents baby him!

THERAPIST: What stopped you?

MELANIE'S ANGRY PART: She won't let me! Every time I'm about to say something, she shuts me down!

This part seems to be talking about another part who inhibits anger.

THERAPIST: Who shuts you down?

Asking a question about this part-to-part relationship

MELANIE'S ANGRY PART: [*A long pause.*] Her mother. But Melanie shuts me down too!

THERAPIST: Want to talk with Melanie about that?

MELANIE'S ANGRY PART: I want her to *listen* to me. I want her to *stop being so scared*!

THERAPIST: Of you?

MELANIE'S ANGRY PART: Of everybody—she can't be around anger at all. She shuts me up and lets other people walk all over her to make sure no one is ever angry! I shout. But even that doesn't do any good!

THERAPIST: I appreciate you sharing this. Would you stand by while I check in with Melanie to see if she's listening to our conversation?

Appreciating the target part and asking it to unblend

MELANIE'S ANGRY PART: [*Nods.*] Okay.

THERAPIST: Melanie, can you shift back? [*She nods.*] Did you hear all that?

MELANIE: I did!

THERAPIST: What is this part talking about?

Supporting part-to-Self relational understanding and insight

MELANIE: That part that is afraid of upsetting everyone, especially my mother.

THERAPIST: Okay. How do you feel toward the angry part now?

MELANIE: I'm appreciating it.

THERAPIST: Ask if it's willing to connect with *you* directly now. [*She nods.*] Share your appreciation, Melanie, and anything else important.

Direct access helps clients notice blended parts and vice versa, which is the beginning of a relationship. An introduction through direct access helps wary protectors feel safer and more connected, smoothing the shift to insight so the client's Self, the primary force for healing, can step in.

Implicit Direct Access	Explicit Direct Access	Insight
The client: • Isn't conscious of the part • Thinks and feels like the part • Is talking to the therapist • Is blended with the part	**The client:** • Is able to partially unblend • Is conscious of a part • Invites the part to blend • Hears the part and the therapist's Self talk	**The client:** • Is conscious of a part • Is inwardly focused • Can access their Self • Is able to unblend from the part
The Self of the therapist: • Talks directly with a part • Doesn't identify it as a part • Gets to know the part	**The Self of the therapist:** • Asks to talk to the part directly • Gets to know the part • Checks back with the client's Self	**The Self of the client:** • Listens to the part • Validates the part's feelings and good intentions • Facilitates the part's healing

Unburdening: The Healing Protocol of IFS Therapy

Once a protector like Melanie's angry part permits the client's Self to access a wounded exile, the following steps, which are designed to meet relational needs, can occur:

1. **Unblending and witnessing:** Exiles need someone kind, concerned, and compassionate (i.e., the Self) to witness their experience. Therefore, at this step the therapist (1) helps a protector part unblend, (2) guides the client to notice the part through the eyes of Self (with curiosity and, if possible, compassion), (3) guides the part to notice the client's Self, and (4) invites the part to tell or show its story to the client's Self in whatever way it wants.

2. **Rescripting:** Often, exiles need a loving, empowered witness to help them with a distressing situation from their past. To do so, the Self comes into the scene and gives the exile whatever help it needed in the past. This allows the exile to "redo" the situation so it can finally leave the past. We call this corrective experience a *do-over* or *rescripting*.

3. **Retrieval:** As soon as the exile is satisfied, the client's Self can help it leave the past and come to the present or go to a fantasy place that the part chooses. If the present is conflict-filled or dangerous, the exile may choose a fantasy place that the Self can visit.

4. **Unburdening ritual:** Here, exiles are invited to release extreme feeling states and let go of toxic identity beliefs (*I am . . . too much, too little, defective*, and so on) through a ritual that can involve one of the five elements (earth, wind, fire, air, water).

5. **Invitation:** Once an exile has unburdened, we ask it to invite in qualities or traits that it may want or need in the future, such as play, fun, freedom, and love.

6. **Integration:** Finally, to release protective parts from their extreme jobs and from a focus on the past, we make sure they've witnessed the exile's transformation, ask if they are ready to change roles, and inquire about their interests: *What would call to you if you didn't have to do this job anymore?*

These steps encompass the heart of *IFS health therapy*, the application of IFS treatment to physical health problems, which emphasizes the release of physical manifestations of burdens that affect the mind-body. We'll discuss these steps in greater detail in chapters 5 through 7.

The therapeutic aim of IFS is straightforward. However, the route can be circuitous. From the perspective of protectors, people (especially grown-ups) are not trustworthy and life has been unsafe, so they are understandably wary. The body, which is a central player in this post-trauma drama, can become a battleground. Physical trauma can lodge exiles in one place in the body. Managers can use the body to frighten and inhibit bolder, more rebellious parts. Firefighters can attempt to soothe the body and silence other parts with highly effective means that exact long-term costs and damage the body. For example, vomiting—a firefighter's way of soothing shame and fear about body weight—erodes tooth enamel, causing decay.

A damaged body can require a great deal of care, and sometimes outside intervention, to heal and function again. When protective parts insist that they can't forgo a damaging habit, perhaps for cultural reasons, the client's Self can patiently explore and intervene. In any case, exiles can be untangled from the body, and the mind-body is mutable. Most everything can shift. Our job is to be curious, compassionate, patient, and convincing. The job of the client's Self is to connect with the exile, witness its losses, validate its worth, challenge past insults, soothe its distress, and act on its behalf.]

[CHAPTER 2]

How Trauma and Shame Get Under Our Skin

Fear, shame, maladaptive guilt, unrelieved anger, helplessness, despair—these are the emotional building blocks of what the medical world calls *stress*, by which they mean the biology of alarm. In IFS, we call these extreme, stuck feelings, thoughts, and mind-body responses *burdens*. As we explain in detail in the passages that follow, we are all born with a biological alarm system. Ideally, when we experience stress, the threat eventually passes, the alarm shuts off, the mind relaxes, the body recoups, and safe social connectivity reigns. But when the body's alarm system never turns off because the stress is persistent, it molds the brain into a "landscape of limitations" (Rediger, 2021, p. 282) and wears the body out, making us more vulnerable to illness and disease. Internalized stress—in other words, *chronic stress*—builds an ongoing, body-wide response that continues throughout our lives. In this section, we explain what stress costs our integrated system of body and parts.

Adverse Experiences Lead to Burdens

As a result of the groundbreaking Adverse Childhood Experiences (ACE) Study (Felitti et al., 1998) and the studies that followed (Caglayan et al., 2025; Jemiyo et al., 2025; Lin et al., 2021; Sonu et al., 2019; Taylor & Demakakos, 2025), we know that childhood trauma is associated with a high risk of poor health outcomes in adulthood. In particular, the original ACE Study identified the cumulative effects of certain childhood traumas and adversities on morbidity and mortality in adulthood, including sexual abuse, psychological and physical abuse or neglect, parental separation or divorce, household violence, substance abuse, and mental illness. Due to the high volume of research that followed this study, we now have a more nuanced and sophisticated understanding of the long-term effects of childhood trauma and adversity on the mind-body. These effects are not solely determined by the type or number of adverse experiences, but by the magnitude, duration, and timing of the biological and behavioral disruptions that lead to increased risk of chronic illness later in life (Shonkoff et al., 2021).

Additionally, many clients who have experienced trauma have not endured the specific traumas or adversities tracked by the original ACE Study, including school shootings, household or neighborhood violence, institutional devaluation, acts of hate, bullying, and other forms of violence that occur outside the home with non–household members. These experiences may also include highly distressing events that some would not classify as trauma, like painful and frightening medical procedures or a persistently unmet need for more adult support at school, which affect the internal system and the body's health. In IFS health therapy, we listen to parts, hear their formative and ongoing experiences, and learn the ways in which these experiences were biologically and emotionally burdening or encouraged health-harming behavior.

As the ACE Study illustrated, children are exquisitely vulnerable to the judgments—implied, enacted, or spoken—of caretakers, authority figures, older children, and peers. A child who is neglected, criticized, raged at, sexually intruded on, assaulted, or subjected to any other kind of violence will feel devalued, hurt, and ashamed. If no one is around to help the child challenge these insults, they must handle it alone. Most often, they learn to tell themselves a damaging story about why this happened to *them* specifically (*I am bad*). Since kids are self-referential, this response is developmentally appropriate and predictable. They don't have a mature perspective—a bird's-eye view—to inform them that other people are motivated by their own personal fears and needs.

These children are at risk of developing *burdens*, which involve fixed negative feelings (e.g., shame, anger, fear) and toxic self-referential beliefs (e.g., *I'm worthless, I'm defective, I'm unlovable*). A variety of adverse experiences can result in burdens—including verbal abuse, physical abuse, accidents, and acts of nature (not least those resulting from climate change)—and evoke fear and the sense of being tiny and unimportant. But these kinds of insults only become *identity burdens* (Sweezy, 2023) if the recipient views them as factual information about who they are. Identity burdens derive from a personal sense of unworthiness.

In addition to developing negative beliefs about our personal value, we inherit burdens from the systems in our environment: our family (parents, relatives, and ancestors), communities, and institutions. In IFS, we call these *legacy burdens*: burdens that are passed down from someone else's sense of personal unworthiness. A legacy burden may have originated generations up the ancestral line due to ethnic or religious oppression, slavery, war, famine, genocide, violence, natural disaster, lack of essential resources, or some other trauma.

Children can also acquire legacy burdens from explicit and implicit biases that arise in their community and its surrounding social systems. Media, schools, universities, medical systems, religious organizations, businesses, and the government are all institutions that have the power to influence our values and prejudices. They instill unconscious as well as conscious cultural biases about, for example, legitimacy, personal value, and success. As a result, we all have legacy burdens.

Social, Cultural, and Environmental Challenges That Contribute to Burdens

Violence and Trauma

- Bullying and abuse in schools and other institutions
- Medical system trauma (e.g., lack of access, unaffordability, dangerous biases)
- Medical treatment trauma (e.g., undergoing an invasive or life-threatening procedure)
- Witnessing or being in an accident
- Witnessing or being the victim of neighborhood violence
- Witnessing or being the victim of terrorism
- Natural disasters and climate change weather events

Discrimination-Based Violence

- Witnessing or being the victim of racial, sexual, or other forms of harassment or terrorism
- Body shaming that singles out some physical feature
- Religious, ethnic, and other forms of discrimination or terrorism
- Income inequality and systemically reproduced poverty

Structural Discrimination and Injustice Involving Access to Resources

Lack of:

- Clean water and air
- Housing
- Healthcare
- Employment
- Education and childcare
- Access to grocery stores
- Affordable fresh food

Regardless of how challenging the circumstance, protective parts try to ensure our survival by helping us adapt. For example, if our ancestors endured poverty and economic instability, we may have a protector who is penny-pinching and anxious about money, even if we have no reason to worry about finances given our current circumstances. As another example, consider Yuri, a client with high blood pressure and an extremely responsible, stoic part, who learned of his great-grandfather's tragic drowning accident, which also claimed the life of his great-grandfather's oldest son. In the aftermath, Yuri's grandfather, who was the second-oldest child, was forced to step in and support the family at just sixteen years old. The burdens of stoicism and over-responsibility were passed on to Yuri's father, and now to Yuri, all stemming from that tragic accident.

Although these protectors' efforts are a testament to ancestral gifts and personal resilience,* we'll focus for the moment on their costs. Most of us are largely ignorant of the ancestral or cultural origins of our family's and our community's negative beliefs, feelings, or behavioral patterns. We absorb these heavy inheritances without conscious intent, and our protective parts are guided by them without discussion, and most often without any sense of choice. To understand why, let's explore in more detail how identity burdens differ from legacy burdens.

Legacy vs. Identity Burdens

A legacy burden isn't personal. It does not imply that "I am . . . defective, too much, too little, bad, or unlovable," as an identity burden does. Rather, it signals loyalty to parents and ancestors: "My protective parts are there for you—they join with you in being afraid, angry, over-responsible, depressed, anxious, or whatever else troubles you—in the hope that you will be there for me." In family therapy terms, these protectors are *parentified*. Out of loyalty, hope, and need, these protectors reverse roles, parenting challenged caretakers and shouldering ancestral burdens.

Whether burdens have to do with someone's personal identity or their cultural/family inheritance, they affect our bodies and parts, leading to a cascade of physiological effects in the mind-body. Here are some examples of how both identity burdens and legacy burdens can affect us:

- **Chronically activated negative feelings.** These can include:
  - Feelings of fear, shamefulness, and anger
  - Fears about being okay due to loss, abandonment, or other threats to survival
  - Feeling like a burden to caretakers
  - Feeling alone while navigating life and dangerous environments
- **Negative beliefs about the self.** These can include beliefs such as:
  - I'm too much.
  - I'm too little.
  - I'm defective.
  - I'm unlovable.
  - I'm unworthy.
- **Bodily sensations that follow the eruption of negative beliefs.** These can include:
  - Cold, clammy hands
  - Hot or cold flashes
  - Increase in perspiration
  - Restlessness

---

* We inherit gifts in addition to burdens. This includes the gifts of confidence, defiance, community, courage, mutual support, love, and special talents or skills. But that is another story.

- Feeling shaky in the limbs
- Speeding up of the heart
- Feeling off-balance or dizzy
- Feeling sick to the stomach
- Feeling frozen, like a deer in headlights
- Numbness and loss of sensory awareness

- **Internal criticism.** This may be due to:
  - Not being neurotypical
  - Being a poor fit with caretakers (e.g., parents, teachers, other adults)
  - Feeling or being different from family or peers
  - Feeling or being alienated in a dominant culture
  - Having a high-anxiety or low-reactivity temperament
  - Criticism or judgment from others
  - Exploitation or violence from a caretaker
  - Any dangerous or painful experience

Although both identity and legacy burdens are profoundly challenging to the integrity and health of the mind-body, they are different. Legacy burdens are all about staying connected. They often run through multiple generations. Parts may be hesitant to let them go, believing they are the connection to family. In contrast, identity burdens are highly personal, isolating, and inherently disconnecting. This leaves exiles and parentified protectors with opposing agendas. Desperate to disconfirm identity burdens and be accepted for who they are, exiles want change. They want to reconnect relationally inside and out. In contrast, parts carrying legacy burdens, like parentification and self-sacrifice, fear any change to the status quo. They believe their loyalty to this inheritance will counter the exile's feeling of invisibility, unimportance, and rejection. They believe the legacy burden reduces the likelihood of being ignored, shamed, and banished again. Reluctant to be disloyal and release legacy burdens, they can prevent the Self from having contact with exiled parts and interfere with progress in therapy. Accordingly, as we will illustrate, protectors who are first and foremost loyal to challenging or dangerous parents or caregivers may need attention before the exile is able to unburden.

Autonomic Nervous System States and Parts

Many adults with unhealed identity and legacy burdens live in dysregulated autonomic nervous system (ANS) states. That's because burdensome beliefs and stuck feelings, along with the numerous strategies protective parts bring to managing them, push the Self out of the body. Although different trauma models use a variety of terms to define and label autonomic states, the ANS states that we describe here (and refer to throughout this book) include: (1) social engagement, (2) fight or flight, (3) freeze or full shutdown,

(4) fawn, and (5) appease (Porges & Porges, 2023). Of these, only social engagement represents a regulated state where the body feels calm and we experience other qualities of Self—like curiosity, compassion, and connectedness—which allows us to care for ourselves and others.

Importantly, a parent or caregiver who is in a dysregulated ANS state and decentered from their own needs can be hard-pressed to attune with a child's emotional needs. For example, a caregiver who is stuck in *fight-or-flight* mode will often overreact to loud sounds, falls in the playground, and children's quarrels with fear or aggression. The child receives the caregiver's alarm and, according to their temperament and priming, withdraws or becomes aggressive. Similarly, a caregiver who is stuck in a *freeze* or *shutdown* state will be "here-but-not-here" (dissociate) in such situations, which can lead the child to conclude, *I'm not worthy of attention* or *I have to take care of my caretaker.* Finally, caregivers who have learned to maximize safety by using a *fawn* or *appease* response with those in positions of power are limited in their ability to offer support or advocacy for their child. In turn, the child may come to believe, *I have to take care of myself,* and develop their own protective strategies.

Relational adjustments like these that attempt to maximize connection promote insecure attachment styles, which have been linked to poorer health outcomes (Mikulincer & Shaver, 2017). Indeed, while the stress response is an adaptive mechanism that has evolved to help us cope with threats or stressors, it can be maladaptive in certain situations, leading to chronic stress–related health problems.

Illnesses and Health Problems Linked to Insecure Attachment Styles

- Sleep disturbance
- Inflammatory illnesses (e.g., rheumatoid arthritis, ulcerative colitis, Crohn's disease)
- Cardiovascular disease
- Breast cancer
- Chronic pain
- Metabolic syndromes (e.g., diabetes, obesity)
- Gastroesophageal reflux disease (GERD)

Together, these ANS responses contribute to, inform, and influence how our parts behave and respond. In IFS health therapy, we believe that these autonomic states are bidirectionally influenced by genetic and environmental factors, including psychosocial experiences. When these autonomic, genetic, and environmental influences manifest inside us (whether physically, emotionally, cognitively, or behaviorally), we call them *parts* and think of them as having different roles and coping strategies. In other words, parts reflect autonomic states, genes, and environmental influences—past and present.

Note also that these ANS responses are not mutually exclusive. For instance, one part may be in a state of fight or flight, while another part is responding submissively in a state of freeze or fully shutdown. Accordingly, in IFS health therapy, clients may notice more than one part (as well as the Self) responding to a situation in different autonomic states. Similarly, in polyvagal theory Stephen Porges talks about hybrid states, or different nervous system states that can combine. In the language of IFS, states change when parts unblend, which comes with access to their Self and social engagement.

The following handout describes the emotional features, physiological changes, and behavioral characteristics that accompany parts as they are affected by autonomic states. The labels and descriptions of ANS states vary by trauma model and author; we use the Porges and Porges (2023) model. From the IFS perspective, autonomic states affect parts and the body bidirectionally.

Autonomic Nervous System States, Parts, and the Self in the Mind-Body

Social Engagement

The ventral vagal branch of the parasympathetic nervous system dominates.

Emotional characteristics: Increased feelings of safety, patience, calm, capacity for connection, open-heartedness, and qualities of the Self are more available.

Physiological characteristics: Promotes regulation and optimal functioning of organ systems relative to an individual's typical range:

- Heart rate reflects calm, and heart feels open and relaxed
- Breathing is deep, slow, and rhythmic
- Muscles relax in the jaw, neck, shoulders, and back
- Gastrointestinal tract is calm and quiet
- Glucose metabolism returns to baseline
- Immune system and inflammatory response return to baseline

Behavioral characteristics: Communicate safety, sociability, trust, and curiosity to others. Our communication promotes connection. We have greater access to Self-leadership and qualities of the Self, such as friendliness and the capacity for compassionate understanding.

IFS health perspective: The Self is accessible. Self-energy is present. Parts feel safe and allow Self to lead, and they either relax back or have Self-energy flowing through them as they relax and connect.

Fight or Flight

The sympathetic nervous system is active.

Emotional characteristics: Fear, anxiety, anger, impatience, or a combination of these emotions.

Physiological characteristics:

- Increased release of adrenaline and noradrenaline
- Hyperarousal and vigilance
- Increased heart rate, blood pressure, and breathing rate
- Dilated pupils and increased sensitivity to sound
- Mobilization of energy resources (e.g., glucose and fats) for quick energy
- Shutdown of nonemergency functions (e.g., digestion, reproductive processes, growth, prefrontal cortex)

Behavioral characteristics: On alert with vigilance, aggression, or escape behaviors in reaction to a perceived threat.

IFS health perspective: A part is cued by a perceived threat, which can activate a burden—an implicit or explicit memory of pain and fear. The emotional and physiological urges to fight or flee reign.

Freeze (Shutdown)

Parasympathetic nervous system dominates—the dorsal vagal branch takes control and shuts down sympathetic activity, leading to immobility and inaction.

Emotional characteristics: Feeling defeated, helpless, hopeless, overwhelmed, or terrified.

Physiological characteristics:

- Drastic drop in heart rate and blood pressure
- Shallow breathing
- Muscular weakness or fatigue
- Difficulty focusing or concentrating
- Constriction of blood vessels (feeling cold)
- Tense muscles
- Inhibition of nonessential bodily functions (e.g., poorer digestion, growth, immunity, reproduction, complex thought)

Behavioral characteristics: Increasing immobility, a deer-in-the-headlights reaction, or a tendency to stay still and silent, with reduced responsiveness to other people and events.

IFS health perspective: A part has been cued by an external event, burden, or implicit or explicit memory. Anxiety, fear, and terror take over as the part freezes in a state of dissociation or shutdown.

Fawn*

Combined activation of both the sympathetic fight-or-flight response and the parasympathetic (dorsal vagal) shutdown response.

Emotional characteristics: Caution, disconnection, fear, hopelessness, or terror, as well as a need to feel safe and connected.

Physiological characteristics:

- Simultaneous fight-or-flight and shutdown stress responses
- Possible elevated heart rate, blood pressure, and muscle tension (fight or flight)
- Possible drop in heart rate and blood pressure and numbness (shutdown)

---

* Fawn and appease are reframed as physiological survival strategies in response to trauma by polyvagal theory, but our understanding continues to evolve in regard to these autonomic states (Porges & Porges, 2023).

Behavioral characteristics: Vigilance, compliance, submissiveness, efforts to please or caretake to achieve safety without the capacity to co-regulate.

IFS health perspective: A manager has been trying to connect without access to the Self. An exile feels scared, alone, or terrified in this state, leading a firefighter to respond with an urge to fight or flee.

Appease

Combined activation of three systems: sympathetic nervous system (fight or flight), parasympathetic nervous system (dorsal vagal), and social engagement system (ventral vagal).

Emotional characteristics: Simultaneous fear, emotional numbness, and capacity for social connectedness and calm.

Physical characteristics:

- Looks calm and present, feels calm and aware, but may alternate between normal arousal, activation, and deactivation as indicated by:
    - Elevated heart rate and blood pressure, perspiration, and thermal fluctuations (feeling hot or cold)
    - Drop in heart rate and blood pressure, constriction of blood vessels, numbness

Behavioral characteristics: Tuned in, calm, supportive of the person in power (e.g., in situations of entrapment such as a hostage, prisoner, or child with unpredictable caregivers). Stays connected by meeting the needs of the other to achieve and maintain safety through co-regulation with the other's autonomic nervous system.

IFS health perspective: An anxious, frightened, and terrified part is shut down, and a part with access to Self-energy manages the potentially threatening situation by sending signals of safety to and co-regulating with the person who has more power.

Positive Stress vs. Toxic Stress

When a child's developmental needs are reasonably fulfilled in relationships at home, at school, and in other environments, the child embodies felt security and attaches safely (Srouf & Waters, 1977), which is the foundation for the emotional and autonomic regulation that supports access to the Self as we grow. *Emotional regulation* refers to our capacity to feel and respond to a range of emotions and return to a state of calm after an upsetting event as parts relax, opening the flow of Self-energy inside. *Autonomic regulation* refers to our capacity to return our physiological systems to their optimal balance and level of functioning as safety is restored, the body recovers, and parts relax after a threat has passed.

Although children don't need perfect environments or relationships to achieve emotional and autonomic regulation, not all stressors are manageable. The frequency, intensity, and duration of a stressor; the age at which it occurs; and the availability of responsive, concerned adults all determine its effects. The National Scientific Council on the Developing Child (2014) has proposed three different categories of stress responses in children—ranging from positive to tolerable to toxic—on the basis of their lasting effects on a child's brain and body:

1. **Positive stress response:** This response is moderate and short-lived; it may involve mild elevations in stress hormone levels and brief increases in heart rate. The natural stress response occurs as a function of the normal ups and downs of life that require moderate adjustment to unfamiliar circumstances; for example, a child might experience this type of response when getting used to a new caretaker or visiting the pediatrician. When children are supported by caring adults, these ordinary life stressors help them become flexible and resilient.

2. **Tolerable stress response:** This occurs as a child's autonomic nervous system becomes more significantly activated, but generally within a limited time period. For example, difficult life experiences like moving to a new town or navigating a death in the family may lead to this more intense stress response. However, if the child has responsive adult support, they can cope with these physiological effects and return to homeostasis, making the stress tolerable.

3. **Toxic stress response:** When a child is exposed to chronic or prolonged stress, and they do not have enough adult support to face the situation, they are unable to turn off their stress response, leading to toxic stress. Children who repeatedly endure difficulties or trauma that is beyond their coping abilities, like maltreatment, community violence, financial hardship, discrimination, or parental depression, become chronically hypervigilant to threat.

Childhood Adversity: Positive, Tolerable, or Toxic Stress	
Determining Factors for Type of Stress	Types of Stress
• Frequency • Intensity • Duration • Age at which the event occurs • Availability of supportive adult help	• **Positive stress response:** The child builds flexibility and resilience by coping with temporary, manageable stress. • **Tolerable stress response:** The child has relational support to cope with serious, acute stress. • **Toxic stress response:** The child experiences chronic, intense activation of their body's stress response systems, causing physiological wear and tear.

Consequences of Chronic Stress

This conceptualization of the stress response underscores the disruptions that can occur when stress is prolonged and long-lasting (Boyce et al., 2021). We know conclusively that experiences in the prenatal period through toddlerhood have lasting effects on both short- and long-term mental and physical health. Children are especially vulnerable to the negative effects of stress at this earliest stage of life because the young brain and immune system are highly plastic and capable of adapting to unique conditions (Boyce et al., 2021; McEwen & Akil, 2020; Shonkoff et al., 2021).

To understand more about the effects of toxic stress, it is important to clarify what happens when the brain initiates the stress response, which is orchestrated among the nervous, endocrine, and immune systems through two main pathways:

1. The sympathetic branch of the autonomic nervous system, the **sympathetic-adreno-medullar (SAM) axis**, releases activating stress hormones called *catecholamines*, primarily adrenaline and noradrenaline, to support the fight-or-flight response. When adrenaline and noradrenaline surge through the body, more blood flows to muscles rather than organs to facilitate a rapid response. Physiological systems mobilize as energy, in the form of glucose, is released into the blood. Nonemergency processes, like gut activity, growth, and reproduction, are all inhibited. These adaptations to stress are called *allostasis*. If the stress is acute and the threat passes, the body returns to normal. If the stress does not end, the body (and our parts) must remain vigilant and sustain these changes. This *allostatic load* or *overload* is "the price the body pays" (McEwen & Akil, 2020, p. 12) for adapting to chronic stress.

2. The **hypothalamus-pituitary-adrenal (HPA) axis** releases stress hormones called *glucocorticoids*, primarily cortisol, to manage metabolic processes necessary for maintaining the ongoing stress response. The HPA axis can kick in relatively soon after the SAM axis, but the HPA axis continues to maintain the production of glucocorticoids as long as we're still under stress. Prolonged exposure

to cortisol can have several side effects, including impaired blood glucose uptake and subsequent elevations in blood sugar levels. In this way, persistent stress responses can overwork and alter our physiological systems, producing proinflammatory effects.

Side Effects of a Prolonged Stress Response

Cortisol, adrenaline, and noradrenaline can contribute to a host of side effects when applied over extended periods, including:

- Immune system dysregulation
- Persistent inflammation
- Neural inflammation and dementia
- Altered glucose metabolism
- Deep abdominal (visceral) fat storage
- Insulin resistance and high blood glucose
- Autoimmune diseases
- Cardiovascular disease
- Increased risk of stroke
- Increased risk of infections
- Depression and anxiety
- Shortening of telomeres (protective ends of chromosome strands)
- Certain forms of cancer
- Disruptions to female reproductive health

In mild to moderately stressed people, the anti-inflammatory effect of glucocorticoids (cortisol) counters the proinflammatory effect of stress. But in chronically stressed people, these anti-inflammatory effects become impaired, allowing "pro-inflammatory effects to go unchecked" (Tong et al., 2023, p. 1). In this way, chronic stress promotes chronic, low-grade inflammation, increases an individual's risk of developing inflammatory diseases, and disrupts the immune system's ability to fight disease and infections. In addition, it increases the likelihood that people will develop depression and anxiety. Since chronic disease, depression, and anxiety are reciprocally influential (Sun et al., 2019), it can be hard to tell which came first.

Chronic Stress and Inflammation

As we've discussed thus far, when stress is short term, the body moves quickly into recovery and returns to homeostasis. In contrast, the effects of chronic stress are cumulative. When the body remains in some degree of autonomic arousal—with our organ systems continually mobilized for danger—it triggers the release of proinflammatory substances called *cytokines*, which increase and promote chronic, system-wide inflammation (McEwen & Akil, 2020). This, in turn, leads to a wide variety of diseases that are collectively the leading cause of death worldwide. While we need the immune system to trigger occasional increases in inflammation to combat infection and injury, ongoing, low-grade inflammation has severe long-term health consequences.

Diseases Linked to System-Wide Chronic Inflammation

Cortisol, adrenaline, and noradrenaline can contribute to a host of side effects when applied over extended periods, including:

- Cardiovascular disease
- Cancer
- Depression
- Osteoporosis
- Insulin resistance
- Type 2 diabetes mellitus
- Chronic kidney disease
- Nonalcoholic fatty liver disease
- Autoimmune diseases (e.g., rheumatoid arthritis, lupus, psoriasis, psoriatic arthritis)
- Neurodegenerative disorders (e.g., Parkinson's disease, Alzheimer's)

The effects of stress-induced inflammation are perhaps most obvious in the relationship between the gut and brain. If you have treated someone with performance anxiety or experienced it yourself, you may know that intense anxiety can prompt a "gut-wrenching" attack of nausea or a need to dash to the bathroom. Chronic inflammation can affect our gut's microbiome, which contains trillions of microorganisms, bacteria, viruses, and fungi spread throughout the gastrointestinal (GI) tract (Sonnenberg & Sonnenberg, 2016). These organisms influence our behavior (i.e., parts) in addition to our metabolism, nutrition, and immunity.

When beneficial gut bacteria thrive—offering us nutrients and services that stimulate the immune system, break down toxins, fend off pathogens, digest fiber, and synthesize micronutrients like B vitamins and vitamin K, amino acids, and much more—the ecosystem of our gut is able to maintain balance. However, psychological stress can disrupt the function and delicate balance of the gut, causing symptoms like increased sensory sensitivity of the GI tract, abdominal pain, altered motility, and leaks in the gut's protective lining that keeps toxins out of the bloodstream. That's because chronic stress dysregulates the HPA axis, leading to sustained elevations in cortisol levels. Excessive cortisol, in turn, affects the gut microbiome, enteric nervous system, and immune system, altering microbial composition and contributing to inflammation such as inflammatory bowel disease (Ge et al., 2022).

IFS Stress-Symptom Cycle for Inflammatory Bowel Disease

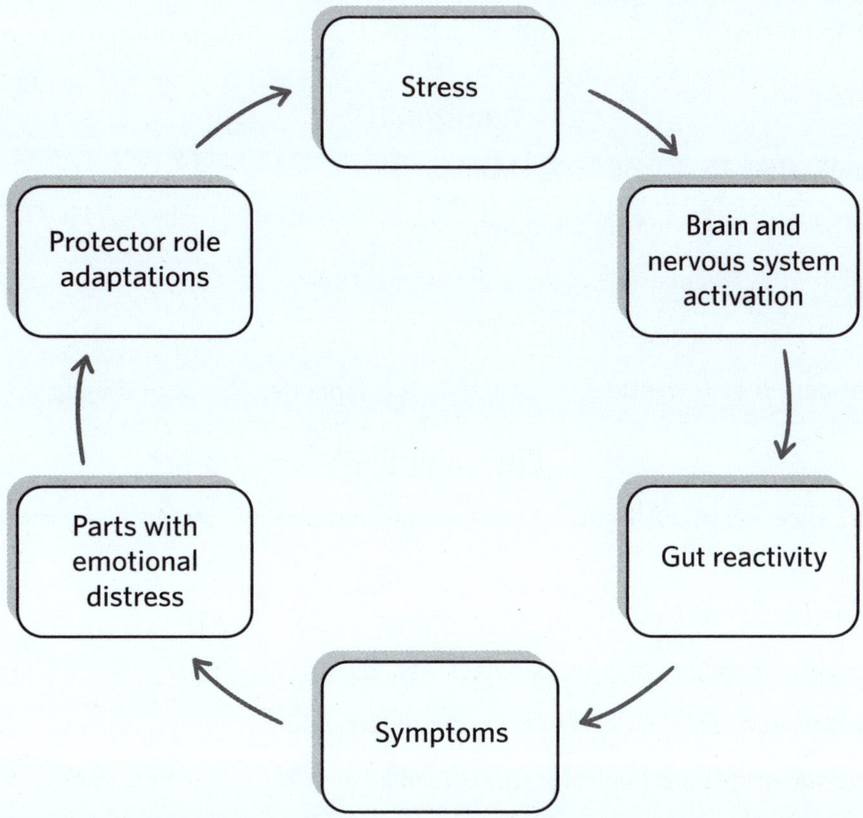

In addition to inflammatory bowel disease, stress-induced inflammation increases the risk of depression and anxiety as well as metabolic disorders like insulin resistance, cardiovascular disease, and autoimmune conditions (Herselman et al., 2022; Kasarello et al., 2023). Collectively, alterations in the gut–brain axis promote changes in cognitive function, emotion regulation, behavior, and stress resilience—and influence parts in turn. While autonomic arousal is an adaptive physiological response to danger in the short term, it causes our mind-body to undergo significant physical wear and tear (allostatic load) over the long term. The following handout describes several of the common symptoms of allostatic load.

Signs and Symptoms of Allostatic Load

Allostatic load: The cumulative health effects of the body's adaptation to chronic stress

Emotional

- **Anxiety/depression:** Persistent worry, sadness
- **Irritability:** Quick to anger, easily offended
- **Anger:** Persistent dysregulation, anger, and high reactivity
- **Loneliness:*** Perceived social isolation
- **Hypervigilance:** On edge, restless, unable to relax, expecting threat or danger

Physiological

- **Sleep disturbance:** Insomnia, frequent awakenings, disrupted sleep cycle, nightmares, vivid dreams
- **Appetite changes:** Eating to self-soothe, overeating, loss of appetite
- **Fatigue:** Persistent exhaustion, physical inactivity, low energy
- **Muscle tension:** Frequent pain in jaw, neck, shoulders, head
- **Gastrointestinal symptoms:** Poor digestion, bowel discomfort, diarrhea, constipation
- **Cardiovascular:** Increased blood pressure, heart rate, disease risk (e.g., heart failure, arrhythmia, arterial plague, aortic aneurysm)
- **Immunity:** Overactivity (allergies and autoimmune disease) or underactivity (more infections)

Behavioral

- **Impaired functioning:** At work, school, or home; in ordinary tasks and social relationships
- **Costly coping strategies:** Substance abuse, health-compromising habits, inner shaming
- **Social:** Withdrawal, avoidance, isolation
- **Difficult to diagnose symptoms:** Unexplained physical complaints, frequent medical visits, avoidance of activities that trigger discomfort

Psychological

- **Cognition:** Poor concentration, forgetfulness, confusion, overwhelm, indecision
- **Cognitive distortions:** Mental filtering, all-or-nothing thinking, catastrophizing
- **Hopelessness:** Pessimism, negative projection, negativity bias

* Loneliness has been shown to mediate the link between social isolation and cardiac distress and disease (Sharif-Nia et al., 2025) and to impact brain as well as cardiac health (Cené at al., 2022).

Inborn Internal Stress

Although stress is often caused by external factors, many of which are beyond our control, some personalities (i.e., configurations of parts) and temperaments leave us more vulnerable to health risk. For example, a cluster of personality traits like moodiness, self-consciousness, and anxiety—often referred to as neuroticism—has been linked to cardiovascular disease (Mahmood et al., 2023; Turiano et al., 2018). Cynicism has also been associated with greater mortality from coronary heart disease, cancer, and stroke (Weiss et al., 2020).

Similarly, some bodies and brains are born with certain disabilities—or acquire disabilities due to injury, aging, or hardship (Cree et al., 2018)—that make us more vulnerable. This can include difficulty with hearing, vision, cognition, mobility, and self-care. In addition, stigma, inequity, and negative bias from the dominant culture—often directed toward those with disabilities or differences like neurodivergence—can amplify these vulnerabilities, burdening our parts and promoting social isolation, ultimately affecting health. Indeed, people with autism experience a greater likelihood of health complications and reduced life expectancy compared to the general population (Bishop-Fitzpatrick & Kind, 2017). Individuals with disabilities are also twice as likely to struggle with depression, asthma, diabetes, stroke, obesity, and poor dental health (World Health Organization, 2023).

In the same vein but more optimistically, IFS asserts that we are born with parts who are particularly vulnerable to dangerous experiences, but they can mend in relationship with the Self inside and with the Self of others outside. Although we can't sort external and internal stressors from genetic factors easily, or untangle the effects of environment from disability and physical injury, these complications are not an obstacle to IFS health treatment. Rather, we can discover the effects of historical injury on the body by befriending the client's internal system and tracking their story.

For example, Tina, a cisgender Dominican American woman in her 40s with a family history of type 2 diabetes, had recently been told that her blood sugar (glucose), triglycerides (a type of fat found in the blood and stored in fat cells), blood pressure, and LDL (bad) cholesterol levels were elevated, indicative of *metabolic syndrome*—a cluster of health conditions that increase the risk of developing cardiovascular diseases and type 2 diabetes. In previous years, Tina's blood glucose, LDL cholesterol, and triglyceride levels had been elevated but not extreme. Her acute stressors were manageable, and although her insulin levels were mildly to moderately elevated, they were stable. But with the COVID-19 pandemic came prolonged, intense stressors. Suddenly, she and her kids were isolated and had to spend hours every day at home doing school and work online. She was afraid for them, her elderly parents, and her husband, who was away on a military deployment.

In addition, the pandemic evoked memories of loss and stress from her childhood, when her family immigrated to the United States from the Dominican Republic. To soothe and distract herself, she stayed up late at night eating snacks and watching TV. Over time, several physical symptoms developed, including muscle tension, a spate of minor infections like cold sores, changes to her menstrual cycle, repeated vaginal yeast infections, constipation, and sleep disturbance. By the time Tina was able to see her doctor in person again, her lab tests revealed a list of rising concerns, all of which signaled metabolic syndrome. Since Tina suspected the culprits were stress along with changes in her exercise and eating habits, she decided to try IFS health therapy.

In IFS health therapy, we listen for indicators in the client's self-report that parts are dealing with ongoing stress (and subsequent stress responses). In Tina's case, her chronic stress resulted from external and internal sources, like the pandemic, her trauma history, and some inherited familial burdens that developed due to racism and the challenges of immigration. Self-soothing with comfort food and distracting with TV exacerbated her already dysregulated autonomic nervous system and HPA axis (which, as we discussed earlier, promotes the release of cortisol and proinflammatory substances). Long-term exposure to cortisol, a possible motivating force in Tina's nightly stress eating, can cause excess abdominal fat (known as *visceral fat* in the medical world) and the release of proinflammatory substances and hormones that interfere with metabolism. This fat affects how cells respond to insulin and how they adsorb glucose for energy in addition to affecting blood glucose levels (Sharma et al., 2022). This complicated interplay between the biology of stress, adaptations in metabolism, and behavioral reward systems contributed to Tina's food cravings, food intake, and weight gain.

Prolonged stress was clearly a risk factor for Tina's escalating health issues. Her therapist wanted to find out which of Tina's parts had been affected by the metabolic changes and which parts, if any, had been active in promoting the conditions that caused the metabolic changes. Burdens and stressors (inside as well as out) affect our health, in part, because they affect the behavior of our parts. Parts will use whatever is available to do their job—even if it comes at a cost to our health. If the situation is ongoing and dire, like the pandemic, they will persist despite rising costs.

"Lifestyle Factors" of Parts Affecting Health

- **Sleep-wake cycle (diurnal rhythm):** When and how well we sleep
- **Social relationships:** Whether we are connected or lonely, trusting or reactive
- **Daily physical activity:** How much we sit, move, and work
- **Nutrition:** How and what we feed our body
- **Self-care and balance:** How well we relate to and meet the needs of our mind, body, and spirit

Whether a stressor is current or continues from childhood (or both), our brains and bodies—including the autonomic nervous system, other interdependent physiological systems, and our internal family system—adapt in ways that that can be costly. Tina's experience illustrates how the brain and body adapt to circumstances that begin even before we're born, as well as how parts of the internal family interact with interrelated organ systems to affect health. Tina's story is one of hardship and resilience. As we discuss how to conduct an IFS health therapy assessment in the next chapter, we continue with her story.

[CHAPTER 3]

IFS Health Therapy Assessment

Introducing the IFS Health Therapy Approach

In IFS health therapy, we are continually assessing the client's mental and physical states. First, we listen and learn. What is this client's presenting problem? What are they willing to hope for from therapy at this point? We couple listening with open-ended questions about their priorities and current circumstances, and we mirror back their answers. We also ask if we can share information and coordinate care with other healthcare providers. At the same time, we assume that while certain parts of the client are speaking up at the start, others will be hanging back or actively kept out of the conversation. A reluctance to disclose important negative experiences and beliefs at the outset of therapy is common and understandable. Some people will readily talk about humiliating, frightening ordeals; others will not. Some will share information about childhood, relationships, and, if applicable, a family history of trauma, but others will be more cautious. All of this information is relevant, so we keep assessing as we go.

In IFS health therapy, as with IFS in general, we want to talk with clients about their parts—what they believe, what they do, what they want, whom they protect, and so on. But we just listen and get curious at the outset. We assume we are hearing from a part—usually the part who brought the client to therapy, but sometimes a part who is reluctant to be in therapy. We address this part directly, sticking with the client's choice of language and using second-person pronouns ("What brings you to therapy?") at first. As they talk, we notice our parts as well as theirs. As discussed in chapter 1, IFS calls this mode of communication implicit direct access. If we were to use explicit direct access instead, we would speak to the part about the client in the third person.

The following vignette continues Tina's story and illustrates how to begin therapy by listening to and talking with one part and then introducing parts language when the opportunity arises. Before coming to therapy, Tina knew she had a genetic predisposition for metabolic syndrome because of her mother's medical history. She also knew she wasn't doomed to get diabetes or have a heart attack, and she was motivated to take action. Nonetheless, she felt daunted when her doctor suggested steps like changes in diet, exercise, and, if possible, weight loss to reduce belly fat. Although Tina's manager fixer part was eager to improve her health, the reactive firefighter who helped her cope with loneliness and fear by snacking and watching TV late into the night rebelled. In response, the manager became even more critical. Until the Self can lead and exiles feel better, proactive and reactive protectors will continue vying for control.

Medically Prescribed Behavior Change and Protector Polarization

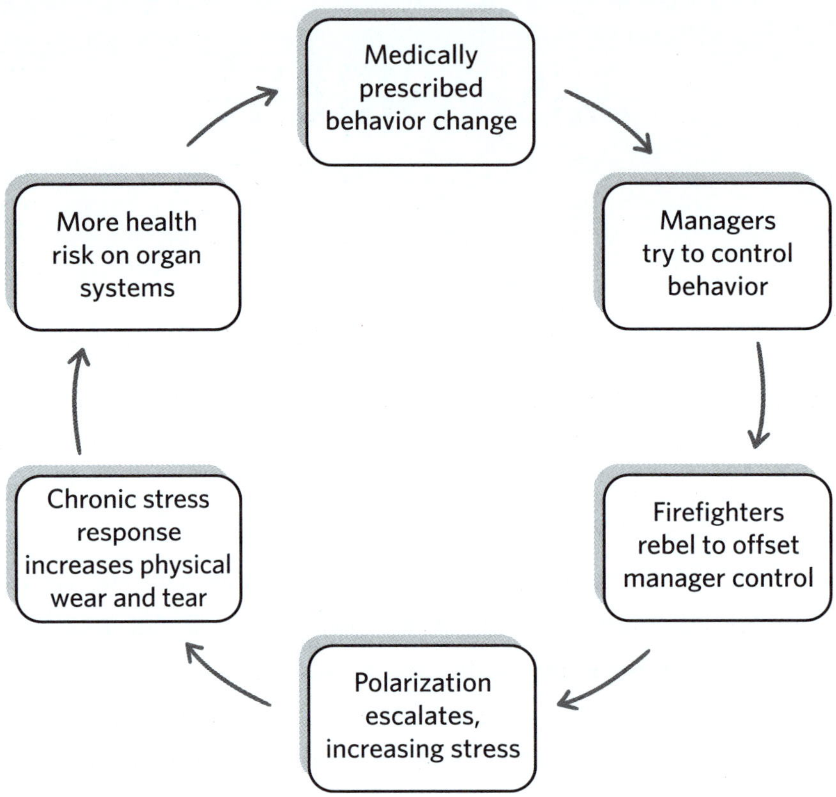

- A critical, shaming manager tries to enforce lifestyle changes to decrease health risk.
- A firefighter rebels to cope with stress, illness, and unhealed burdens like shame.
- The manager and firefighter escalate in relation to each other, becoming ever more extreme.
- Their conflicting coping behaviors add stress to the body.
- Autonomic arousal continues as their conflict escalates, increasing allostatic load and producing more wear and tear on the body.
- Chronic stress and escalating coping behaviors (e.g., alcohol, drugs, overeating) increase health risks.

Since Tina's worried, highly critical manager believed therapy would help her "stay on track" with the doctor's suggestions, it tried to recruit the therapist as an ally. While we do not take sides when proactive and reactive parts polarize, we know both sides mean well and can, with encouragement, become partners in prevention and healing.

In this session, Tina came to therapy blended with this critical part, who held her responsible for the increasing insulin resistance. This part constantly shamed and blamed her. The therapist noticed and spoke to this part directly without mentioning it as a part.

Therapist: When we spoke on the phone, you said that your insulin resistance had skyrocketed during the pandemic when you were working long hours without enough downtime or sleep. Is that right?

The therapist says "you" but is addressing a part. This is implicit direct access.

Tina: That's right. It was so intense! My kids were doing school online and I was worried about my parents. I stayed up late to get some time to myself—and, boy, did I eat. I know I have to change my eating habits. I know it's how I got through the pandemic, but it has to stop! This is my fault.

Therapist: You blame yourself and your eating habits. [*Tina nods.*] Are you concerned that I might judge you too?

Again, rather than switching to parts language, at this point, the therapist keeps addressing the part with the second-person pronoun "you" as if it were the client.

Tina: Well, why wouldn't you judge me? My diet is obviously the problem.

Therapist: But I don't think it's your fault, Tina.

Tina: You don't know how much time I spend in front of the TV at night eating after I get everyone to bed. And I used to smoke! [*She shakes her head.*] I'm out of control.

Therapist: I have a different view. You have *parts* who are dedicated to doing whatever they can to help you with chronic stress, even if it harms your health.

Now the therapist is switching to parts language and addressing the positive intent of parts who engage in health-harming habits.

Tina: What do you mean?

Therapist: By the word *parts*? [*Tina nods.*] I mean you're normal. We all have conflicting opinions and agendas at times. It's a sign of what I call "parts" or "subpersonalities." One part of you eats to feel better when you're exhausted and overworked, and then another part worries about the health consequences of self-soothing that way. Do you hear both of them?

Inner polarities are often a good opportunity to point out the existence of parts.

Tina: You're saying that a part of me is helping me out with nighttime eating and TV watching?

Therapist: Of course, eating that way contributes to the undesirable outcome of higher blood glucose and cholesterol, so the idea that part is trying to help in this way may sound strange. But notice that the part intends to lower your stress. Dedicated parts will do whatever they can to help us cope in the moment.

Tina: Yeah, but everyone else dealt with stress during the pandemic, and not everyone was foolish enough to bring on diseases that run in their family. I'm so ashamed! I'm mad at myself. Why wouldn't you judge me?

The critical part is still talking.

Therapist: I get why you might expect to be judged. Our culture sells self-soothing with comfort food and then criticizes the effects, especially in women. We're all subject to this bias. If you sense it in me, please let me know. Here in our time together, I want us to talk freely without judgment. I don't want any culturally burdened parts of me to judge you about weight or anything else.

The therapist addresses culturally based biases that contribute to legacy burdens.

Tina: [*Nods thoughtfully.*] I appreciate you saying that. I don't think I sensed any judgment coming from you. But it does happen a lot.

Therapist: I know. The diet culture and judgments about how we look—our size, shape, and color—wait for us at every turn. I'm honestly not sensing that kind of judgment in me right now either. But if anything like that comes up, we can talk about it. We all are steeped in these biases. Our parts try their best to cope, mine included.

The therapist asserts the universality of parts and invites transparency.

Tina: Thank you. I'm not used to hearing that, but it helps. You really think snacking at night is an effort by some part of me to lower stress?

Therapist: I do. But don't take my word for it. Let's ask your parts directly what they're trying to do for you.

In this session, the therapist introduced Tina's inner critic to the nonpathologizing perspective of IFS health therapy: that all parts have good intentions, even if their short-term protective responses have a cascading negative effect on the mind-body. Over time, the therapist will share more specific information regarding the cumulative effects of chronic stress and persistent episodic stress on organ systems, which can lead to a host of health problems and stress-related diseases. Although genes play a role in many illnesses, parts can play a role in any illness. We know, for example, that eating and activity habits (i.e., the behaviors of parts) can reduce or increase the expression of genes for insulin resistance and other conditions related to metabolic syndrome through epigenetic change (Maude et al., 2021). Indeed, parts can and do affect health. This idea may alarm some clients, especially if:

- Their illness is related to behavior, like smoking, physical inactivity, or diet, that comes with a shaming cultural bias or health-related stigma (Dolezal & Bynum, 2024).
- A medical professional or some other authority figure referred them to therapy, either because they understood the connection between illness and chronic stress or because they could not reach a medical diagnosis and concluded that the problem was likely emotional.
- Their identity burdens (e.g., *I'm bad, I'm worthless*) from past experiences provoke self-criticism and stoke the fear of being shamed again by other people.

Accordingly, the therapist also needed to address Tina's fear of being blamed. If the presenting illness can be related to the way the client's parts are behaving, we have to address the client's own self-blame while also not forgetting the realistic fear that the client may be shamed and blamed by other people. Here, the therapist broached pervasive cultural biases about weight, size, and race and let Tina know that these subjects weren't taboo in their relationship.

Practitioners of IFS know that parts—our own included—can be quick to engage in bias if it serves a protective agenda, and they may behave badly or simply be oblivious to the feelings of other people. The behavior is reprehensible, but the part actually has good intentions and is simply stuck in an extreme job. It's understood in IFS that protectors need to be helped rather than exiled, and that extreme behavior, including prejudice, is what we call a *trailhead*, or a guide to which part needs attention first.

The Fear of Shame and Blame

When clients are stuck in a shame cycle, they are primed to view themselves negatively as well as to accept criticisms from others (Sweezy, 2023). Additionally, therapists have their own burdens and may be primed to judge behaviors that contribute to health problems. Accordingly, IFS therapists who work with clients to heal physical health problems are trained to address personal burdens and be aware of parts in themselves who are biased about any of the following:

- Eating habits
- Activity level and exercise
- Dietary habits and nutrition
- Sleep habits
- Smoking and substance use
- Behavioral addictions
- Sexual behaviors
- Physical features (e.g., race, weight, ability)

Since all parts have good intentions (Schwartz & Sweezy, 2020), the maladaptive thinking and behavior of protective parts makes sense once we hear their motives. We can enter the process of assessment with positive regard for all parts and a particular appreciation for the creativity of the protectors who have helped the client to function during tough times. The IFS assessment is explicitly nonpathologizing and guides the client to begin forming relationships with these parts.

Addressing Shaming and Blaming

Bring kindness and a firm but light touch to parts who shame and blame the client about illness and health risk behaviors. In Tina's case, the illness was metabolic syndrome and the behavior was eating in response to stress.

1. **Acknowledge reasons for concern** to the critical part: "Eating behavior can contribute to insulin resistance and cardiovascular disease."
2. **Validate the part's concern:** "It makes sense that you're concerned about the high blood glucose levels, hypertension, and elevated triglycerides."
3. **Place the behavior in the context of stress or trauma** in the client's life: "But even parts who engage in behaviors that can be destructive for the body intend to help with ongoing stressors like the pandemic, overwork, or lack of rest."
4. **Appreciate the part** who is trying to meet a need or who feels responsible: "Dedicated parts will do whatever works in the short run."
5. **Offer possibility and make room for skepticism:** "But don't take my word for it. Let's hear from your parts directly and find out what they're trying to do for you."

After this first session, Tina and her therapist had enough information to start treatment. First, Tina wanted to manage her blood glucose and LDL cholesterol levels so she could avoid type 2 diabetes and coronary artery disease. This would involve either stabilizing her current levels or, if possible, reducing her insulin resistance and LDL cholesterol. Since stress is an identified factor in both insulin resistance and type 2 diabetes (Sharma et al., 2022; Yaribeygi et al., 2022), as well as in elevated LDL cholesterol (Satoh et al., 2022) the question became: Would reducing her stress, fear, and the physiological wear and tear on her mind-body help lower her insulin resistance and cardiovascular risk? We could not predict, but we could find out.

Second, Tina identified several behavioral changes that could move the needle on metabolic syndrome, like increasing her physical activity, eating fewer and more nutritious calories, and reducing stress. She also identified the polarized protective parts who were contributing to her cycle of chronic stress: one group of parts stayed up late, watched TV, and snacked to cope with stress, while another group of parts were concerned about Tina's health and shamed the stress-eating part. To diagnose a problem in IFS health therapy, we must identify the parts who are caught in a chronic stress cycle. Both internal and external stressors affect parts through:

- **Dysregulation:** This occurs when ongoing sources of stress overwhelm the client's coping capacity. Persistent anxiety, fear, and physiological dysregulation (e.g., chronic states of fight or flight, freeze or shutdown, fawn or appease) affect the body, interdependent organ systems, and the internal system of parts.
- **Costly roles and coping strategies:** Coping parts in extreme roles are attached to temporary fixes that work quickly but bring negative health consequences down the road. Extreme coping

strategies can include leveraging health symptoms to gain needed attention or avoid overwhelming responsibilities. The most common quick-fix option—an addictive process—affects work, play, physical activity, sleep, eating, social support, and relationships.

In chapter 4, we'll talk about the chronic stress cycle in more detail and discuss how to use it to explore the biological, psychological, and social roots of the client's health problems.

What We Listen for and Talk About in IFS Health Therapy

In addition to listening for shame and blame, as well as stressful experiences that can have a negative effect on parts and the body, we also listen for a legacy of family trauma or chaos. A history of dysregulated family, cultural, and social systems can cause ongoing autonomic dysregulation. Protectors work hard to handle or combat the dysregulation in their environment—and the more pain these external systems inflict, the more they look outward for help and solutions. While this makes sense, instability in the client's *own* internal system is the driving force behind their distress. Internal processes are the engine of despair and need to be addressed first. Despair arises from, on one hand, disconnection from the Self, and on the other hand, from past frightening, shaming, or physically painful experiences that live on inside and are easily evoked by similar experiences in the present.

To intervene when the past keeps intruding on the present, clients must ultimately do what IFS calls a *U-turn*, which means they will need to focus inside and help parts and the body before they can effectively tackle problems with external people or systems. Some protectors fear the U-turn at first, but as they experience *co-regulation*, the calming that comes from relational connection and collaboration in therapy, they tend to grow willing. In the following dialogue about control, Tina takes her first step toward a U-turn.

Therapist: Do you have any questions so far about IFS therapy and its potential for improving your health concerns?

Tina: It sounds like you might be able to help me change some of my behavior—what you call a part—but it also sounds like there's more to this than me being accountable.

Therapist: There is. This therapy can help with the behavior of parts who contribute to the problem of insulin resistance, high blood pressure, and so on. But we won't try to control them. It's not polite and it doesn't work.

Tina: Oh, well! I know trying to control my eating is a losing battle. But what else is there?

Therapist: First, we'll talk with the critic who's so worried. Then, we'll get to know the part who does the stress eating.

Tina: [*Laughs.*] You mean I can't just clobber the stress eater?

The Initial Goals of IFS Health Therapy

As Tina's session proceeded, the therapist shifted from talking with Tina's critical part to explaining the idea of parts and engaging her curiosity (a crucial quality of the Self). When the therapist went on to assert that protective parts have good intentions, it took Tina by surprise. Could the part who eats in the night *really* mean to help? This surprise facilitated another bit of unblending, allowing Tina to step away from the critical (formerly fully blended) part's perspective on its rival, the stress-eating part. She was seeing the stress-eating part in a new light. When parts unblend, we access a uniquely comforting and powerful state of mind, and changes also occur in the body. We may observe more receptivity, softening, curiosity, connection, and possibly even playfulness, humor, or other expressions of creativity. In Tina's case, the therapist watched Tina grow more relaxed and thoughtful, and sit back in her chair. Her critical part was taken off guard by the therapist's counterintuitive perspective on nighttime eating, while her stress-eating part was startled to feel understood and appreciated for the first time. By shaking things up in this way, we help polarized parts out of their calcified viewpoints and open the door to new possibilities.

Thus far, the therapist had used the following steps to facilitate unblending with Tina:

1. Implicit direct access at the outset of treatment
2. Introducing the word *part* and noting Tina's receptivity
3. Speaking of parts with positive regard and describing their good intentions
4. Observing changes in Tina's insistence on self-blame, her overall perspective, and tension in her body

As the session progressed, the therapist used the concept of the Self to further facilitate the process of unblending. She also made connections between parts, the mind-body, the stress response, and Tina's health problems. The following dialogue shows the therapist helping Tina track parts consciously and notice their physiological impact.

Therapist: Hey! You're really getting this. No clobbering! But seriously, when worried parts relax, our natural capacity for curiosity, calm, and other helpful states of mind comes online.

Tina: You mean if I get to know the part that overeats, I will stop panicking about insulin resistance, weight gain, and other metabolic symptoms?

Therapist: You do need to help the part who's panicking and judges the eating—and also the part who stays up late eating. We can help them both.

Tina: I guess they do both need help if I'm going to make changes.

Therapist: This is normal. Living is a challenge. Our parts help us survive, and then they need help. Now that you're grown up, you can help them. They need you.

Tina: Okay. I have to take this in. Explain again what parts do to my health.

Therapist: Parts live in what I call the mind-body, because the mind and body are intertwined. Parts are affected by your experiences and later by your memories of those experiences. Unresolved emotional injuries and stress from bad experiences will continue to affect your nervous system, stress response, biological processes—like blood sugar levels and glucose metabolism—and your parts. When we help your parts, we help your body, and vice versa.

TINA: I thought my head would explode during the pandemic. Even though I knew overeating was a problem, a voice in my head said, *Screw it. I have to get through this somehow!*

THERAPIST: Yes, the *screw it* part was helping you cope with the stress. [*Tina suddenly looks unhappy and tense.*] What's happening?

TINA: I remember how badly I wanted to escape.

THERAPIST: And now?

TINA: Yeah, now too. No offense. [*They both laugh.*] Coming here I did feel . . . I don't know. Dread?

THERAPIST: We're here to help parts with their dread or stress or whatever they feel. They all deserve relief.

TINA: It's funny, but I'm glad to feel something right now. This is new. I take care of business—I'm great at that. I'm a fixer, not a feeler.

THERAPIST: Sounds like your fixer part jumps in to ward off feelings. But, of course, your parts all have feelings. We can help them share those feelings safely, without overwhelming each other.

The therapist took note of the thoughts, feelings, and behaviors that were typical of Tina's dominant protectors, with the intent of exploring these in future sessions. These included statements Tina made about herself, like her desire to escape, her dread, and her observation that she was "a fixer, not a feeler." With the ultimate aim of improving Tina's metabolic syndrome, these clues would guide the therapist in exploring the interface between Tina's internal and external stressors, her active protectors, and her body.

How We Talk in IFS Therapy

With this session in mind, let's return to the subject of how we talk in IFS health therapy. As mentioned earlier, when a client makes initial contact and at the beginning of the first session, we use implicit direct access to talk with the presenting part, who generally says things like "I feel . . . I want . . . I'm looking for . . ." and so on. We mirror this back using second-person pronouns ("You feel . . . You want . . . You're looking for . . ."). To the client and the outside observer, this looks like regular talk therapy, but from the IFS perspective, the therapist is engaging a part, the one who is trying to set the table for therapy. This leading part is often a proactive protector (a manager) who is trying to recruit the therapist to the cause of improving the client's being and behavior. On the other hand, this part could be a reactive protector (a firefighter) who is wary of—or actively opposing—therapy, or a banished exile who has broken out of jail. Exiles make the client look fragile or collapsing, which is why protectors keep them locked up. We'll show you how to welcome a manager now and get to reactive protectors and exiles later on.

If a client finds that their parts won't interact with them at all—for example, if the part in the lead ignores the client or claims to be the client—the therapist can speak to it as a part and talk to it about the client in the third person (e.g., "I know you're an important part of Tina. You are brave and strong and take the lead a lot. And I hear the stress-eating part annoys and worries you, so I know you're not the only part of Tina. But there's also a Tina who's not a part. Would you like to meet her? She could help."). We will illustrate this option in greater detail in chapter 5.

As in all IFS therapy, Tina's therapist made some judgment calls in the first session, adjusting the pace and introducing new concepts according to Tina's level of comfort with:

- The IFS vernacular
- The concept of parts
- The idea that somatic experiences, feelings, thoughts, and behaviors are how parts show up in the mind-body
- Attending inward (*going inside*) on the body and mind to locate parts

The idea of parts and the language used in IFS can evoke many responses. Some people get confused, disoriented, or uncomfortable; others immediately relate and feel their internal experience is being validated ("I'm always saying part of me feels this and part of me feels that!"). We adjust accordingly. If a client objects to parts language, we can use implicit direct access (e.g., "So when your boss decided to override your decision, you felt angry and wanted to tell him off, but you also thought it would be a mistake to react. I understand both of those responses. Do you?") and then wonder if these *parts* would like help talking it over. We can also translate the client's language—*I sense, I feel, I think, I did*—into parts language. We can always use the client's language to insert the systemic concepts of IFS experientially. For example: "What happens if you . . .

- . . . allow that angry feeling inside without pushing it away?"
- . . . get curious about the mix of thoughts or feelings?"
- . . . tune into the [*symptom, tension, or sensation*] and notice the feelings or thoughts that come up?"

The IFS approach is attuned, respectful, nonpathologizing, and systemic, all of which appeals to most parts. We frame strong emotional reactions and negative thoughts as crucial information, and problematic behaviors as well-intentioned protective coping strategies that are effective in the short run but too expensive over time. In addition, we are not directive about the client's process. They can close their eyes to focus internally or not; they may see their parts or not. We invite them to be curious and learn how their system communicates and what it needs. The client whose mind has been full of strife and fear may need to approach slowly. That's okay. We go at their pace, offering patience, presence, and interest.

Progressing Between Sessions and During Sessions

Once the client has identified their goals, the client and therapist can identify the parts who need attention first and track them session to session. The therapist should keep notes of some kind to support flow and consistency, and some clients like to do this as well. Over time, the client builds relationships with parts related to their illness. On the next page, you will find a simple form, which includes a checklist of descriptors, for tracking parts and their progress efficiently. The form takes note of stressful external events and social interactions as well as feelings, thoughts, beliefs, and symptoms that occurred during the week. It also has space for a brief description of how the session ended and where to pick up in the next meeting.

IFS Health Therapy Tracking Form

Client name: ______________________________ Date: ______________

Symptoms: ____

____

____

Subjective units of distress scale (SUDS):* Physical state __________ Emotional state __________

Changes since last session (physical or psychological): ______________________

____

____

____

Trailhead focus this session: ______________________________

Parts targeted this session: ______________________________

____

____

Check those that applied to this session. With therapeutic support, the client was able to:

- ☐ Identify a trailhead and target part
- ☐ Identify burdens carried in the system
- ☐ Get permission from protectors to work with a target part
- ☐ Help protectors step back
- ☐ Address protector fears, when necessary
- ☐ Offer hope and a positive vision of healing
- ☐ Understand the positive intension of protective parts
- ☐ Establish Self-to-part relationship with ______________________ [*name part*]
- ☐ Get to know a target part
- ☐ Deepen Self-to-part relationship with ______________________ [*name part*]
- ☐ Witness the target part

- ❒ Offer an emotionally corrective experience (a.k.a. do-over)
- ❒ Retrieve the part from the past to present
- ❒ Release burdens from the past (unburdening ritual)
- ❒ Help an exile/target part to invite in qualities or traits needed going forward
- ❒ Integrate a previous "going inside" experience: ______________________________

  ____
- ❒ Set intentions or make commitments with part(s): ______________________________

  ____
- ❒ Focus on the therapeutic relationship
- ❒ Focus on external stressors: ______________________________

  ____
- ❒ Focus on internal stressors:** ______________________________

  ____
- ❒ Respond to implicit direct access
- ❒ Respond to explicit direct access
- ❒ Experience legacy unburdening

SUDS at the end of the session: Physical state ______________ Emotional state ______________

Where did the session end? ______________________________

____

Where does it make sense to pick up next session? ______________________________

____

* Rate the client's SUDS level on a 0 to 10 scale, with 0 being no distress and 10 being extreme distress.

** Internal stressors include negative feelings, thoughts, beliefs, or behaviors that increase internal or external conflict, anxiety, fear, and health risks.

Interfacing with Other Systems and Information Sources

Mental Health Diagnosis

While IFS health treatment does not require a diagnosis, it can help to find parts linked to physical illness. Depression, for example, is associated with many chronic diseases, including cardiovascular, inflammatory, and metabolic diseases, as well as neurological disorders and cancer (Gold et al., 2020; Souama et al., 2023). Similarly, anxiety disorders have been linked to the development of cardiovascular disease, perhaps because of related increases in autonomic dysregulation, inflammation, and blood clotting (Celano et al., 2016).

IFS health treatment understands *Diagnostic and Statistical Manual of Mental Disorders* (*DSM*) diagnoses as aggregate descriptions of how parts tend to behave in response to physical or social threats. Nonetheless, we provide a *DSM* diagnosis when needed to:

- Interface with non-IFS-informed systems like health insurers and hospitals
- Communicate with non-IFS-trained colleagues to coordinate treatment
- Integrate IFS with other models and modalities
- Incorporate research from various fields (e.g., medicine, epigenetics, trauma, affective neuroscience)

In our experience, the most pointedly relevant *DSM* diagnosis for IFS health treatment is often overlooked. It is called "Psychological Factors Affecting Other Medical Conditions." Clients who receive mental health treatment for psychological or behavioral factors that adversely affect a medical condition meet the criteria for this diagnosis if their symptoms are not better explained by other mental health disorders, such as posttraumatic stress disorder (PTSD), some other anxiety-related disorder, or major depression.

Medical Diagnosis

Physical problems can be mysterious, multilayered, and characterized by nonspecific symptoms like pain or redness of the skin. Healthcare providers are trained to identify a disease, condition, or syndrome—that is, give a diagnosis—in order to explain symptoms, determine treatment, and offer a reasonably accurate prognosis. This linear process, which may or may not cite underlying causes and identify how the problem developed, works well for some health issues but not others.

For example, it helped Tina and her IFS therapist identify the factors that contributed to her metabolic symptoms. But this kind of information is not always available. The origin of a medical condition can be elusive, and healthcare professionals in the United States—who are charged with symptom relief and put under constant time pressure, often in settings with scarce resources—may be unable to pursue the question of origins in any case. Providers face a perpetually expanding body of high-quality research on how stressors, including environmental hazards and psychosocial factors like Tina's family history of immigration and social injustice, affect human health (Larson et al., 2017; Vineis & Barouki, 2022), which can be overwhelming to navigate.

By educating ourselves about a client's medical diagnosis, we can help. We can contextualize and we can delve into the effects of interactions between parts, the mind-body, the environment, and life experience. We can identify possible factors that affect health, like the coping behaviors of Tina's protective parts, which ultimately altered how her body metabolized glucose and responded to insulin. Those of us who like reading journal articles can do that—many open access articles are available online—and those of us who have little time can find summaries of various medical conditions from reliable health resources that are regularly updated and published online.

Risk Factors: Genes, Environment, and Parts

The scientific study of the interface between nature (genetics) and nurture (environment) helps us understand the impact of environment on the expression of genes (epigenetics) that affect the functioning of bodily systems and behavior. We make use of this information to:

- Identify key factors affecting the brain and body (e.g., negative beliefs and dysregulation)
- Understand the link between stressful or traumatic life events and their subsequent impact on beliefs, feelings, and behavior (i.e., parts) as well as bodily systems
- Identify any affected, burdened parts (e.g., Tina's lonely exile and her nighttime-snacking protector)
- Reduce the client's shame and self-blame with accurate information (e.g., the physiological impact of stress and trauma)
- Identify desirable changes in the internal social system of parts affecting health (e.g., the extreme role of Tina's stress-eating part)
- Communicate and collaborate with others in the healthcare system who don't think about stress reduction or emotional/physiological dysregulation in terms of parts

Our understanding of the influence of life experience and the environment on genetic predispositions—like the cluster of cardiometabolic conditions that Tina inherited from her mother—continues to expand with genomic research. For example, Tina, like her mother, was at risk for type 2 diabetes, cardiovascular disease, and stroke. Her family history of chronic stress and trauma, including her mother's gestational diabetes before she was born, contributed to Tina's own health risk (McEwen & Akil, 2020; Sharma et al., 2022; Souama et al., 2023). Tina's parts responded to the intense stress of the pandemic in ways that helped in the present but increased her risk for these serious health problems downstream. Nonetheless, her therapist—who had learned that reducing stress and belly fat while increasing good nutrition and activity can all make a difference in the body's response to insulin—was confident that treatment could help Tina's cardiometabolic conditions. Together, they were able to identify a great starting place: the conflict between her stress-eating part and her critical part.

Collaborating with Physicians and Other Healthcare Providers

During the initial assessment process, the therapist will have asked for (and hopefully gotten) permission to contact the client's referring physician. Once both providers have a release, they will communicate. We can't predict whether a physician will have the time and interest to collaborate, but a prior collegial relationship or awareness of mutual benefit helps. In any case, after the first couple of sessions, the therapist will likely have a good sense of how a collaborative relationship with the client's physician would help.

We have worked with physicians or other healthcare providers who spotted underlying emotional factors and were eager to collaborate; we have worked with medical providers who were not aware of what IFS health treatment could offer but were open to new ideas; and we have also treated many clients for physical conditions without coordinating with their medical providers because of various logistic obstacles, including the physician having insufficient time or interest. While collaboration is preferable, its absence will not prevent IFS health therapy from being effective.

Our role as IFS therapists is to facilitate the revival of parts afflicted by trauma and chronic stress who activate or exacerbate symptoms and compromise health—whether or not we collaborate with other healthcare providers. We start by allowing the client to tell their story and name the presenting problem, just as Tina did. In IFS, we assume this storyteller is a part. Tina spoke from a concerned, proactive manager part. As we listen to the presenting part, we think about a system of players who share a desire to be loved and safe but disagree on tactics. They usually come to therapy afraid, unhappy, and in conflict with each other. We aim to help the client notice them and, as much as possible, be noticed by them. This process of unblending sets the stage for parts to have courageous conversations with the client's Self and with each other about the important things in life, inside as well as out (Herbine-Blank & Sweezy, 2021). In the next chapter, we will discuss how relational healing happens in treatment.

[CHAPTER 4]

Setting the Relational Stage

Clients start IFS health therapy with an underlying accumulation of problems that developed due to genes, life experiences, and age—with the prenatal months, early childhood, and adolescence being particularly vulnerable periods (Boyce et al., 2021; Gescher et al., 2018). The impact of stressful circumstances and events varies according to their frequency, intensity, and duration, as well as the availability of relational support during those times. Therefore, what some people can tolerate will be traumatic for others. The IFS health therapist aims to help the client feel better—to get relief from internal and external stress in a way that decreases the need for their biological systems (and their internal family of parts) to adapt in ways that exact a toll on the client's health.

In particular, we aim to help the client's mind-body exit the "disease superhighway" (Rediger, 2021, p. 111). To do so, frightened parts need relational and internal security. We know that once banished parts are reinstated with care through witnessing and unburdening, and once protectors resolve their disagreements, the mind-body moves from "survival mode" to "mending mode." Clients can recalibrate a chronically stressed system by looking at themselves through eyes of a therapist who sees not only their burdens from trauma, loss, and chronic stress, but also their wholeness and goodness. Our job is to support clients as they develop sustainable, satisfying, Self-led relationships with the body and their parts inside, and with other people outside. When their parts feel loved, they can turn off their high-alert "default mode" of fear and shamefulness and recalibrate.

In IFS health treatment, healing is an unfolding, relational process distinct from the idea of a cure. We don't know where the inquiry will take our clients, but we aim for a mind-body outcome that eases symptoms. Helping the client regulate their nervous system and make lifestyle changes can contribute to a cure (Rediger, 2021)—and we have seen cures (the remission of a biological disorder) over the course of IFS health therapy—but cures are rare when it comes to noncommunicable, chronic diseases, and we can't attribute them to therapy. Accordingly, curing is neither our goal nor our measure of success. Rather, we aim to facilitate healing as the client comes to know and care for their protective and vulnerable parts. With compassionate oversight, the client's Self helps exiled parts jettison the myth of shame by revealing their intrinsic worth, which in the process, frees protectors from the onerous, stress-producing job of scolding and shaming. In IFS, the concept of healing encompasses the belief that burdens and the strategies of protective parts obscure the wholeness intrinsic to our nature.

Since the journey of IFS health therapy unfolds daily and transforms life incrementally, it can change the course of chronic illness. As the client experiences more self-compassion and Self-leadership, they feel better and they are more skillful in relationships. This is what we saw in the IFS rheumatoid arthritis study at Brigham and Women's Hospital in Boston (Shadick et al., 2013). The study had two cohorts: One group received rheumatoid arthritis educational materials with follow-up calls, while the other received IFS health therapy in small groups and individual sessions. One of the coauthors of this book, Nancy, was the facilitator of the small intervention groups throughout the study. She noted that the patients' typical stoicism softened as they learned the IFS model, and as they felt compassion for themselves and others they gradually felt better physically and mentally. At the one-year follow-up, this group continued to relate to their parts with compassion (Shadick et al., 2013).

The Overarching Goals of IFS Health Treatment

We plan to help clients feel better and aim to:

1. Stabilize symptoms
2. Slow the biological progression of the client's illness
3. Improve or arrest symptoms as much as possible

These are hopes—and unknowns. While we look for improvement and know that a cure can occur, we don't make promises or assumptions.

IFS Health Therapy: A Relational Healing Process

Our first and primary goal in IFS health therapy is relational healing in the mind-body. Self-leadership is a better option than clients have known to date. It challenges physiological and behavioral adaptations that harm health by (1) identifying and helping parts who are stuck in fear-driven roles that contribute to health problems and (2) promoting emotional and physiological regulation to reduce the wear and tear of chronic stress on the mind (Comeau et al., 2024) and body. To do so, we collaborate with the client and, when possible, involve other treaters, treatment groups (Comeau et al., 2024), and individuals who are in the client's support network. In other words, we attend to both inner and outer relationships.

IFS health therapy emphasizes the importance of relationships to health. Close relationships may be even more important to long-term health than well-known risk factors like smoking, visceral fat, and physical inactivity (Holt-Lunstad et al., 2022; Pietromonaco & Beck, 2019; Pietromonaco & Collins, 2017). In fact, the ongoing, decades-long Harvard Study of Adult Development reveals that satisfying relationships are the most critical factor in long-term health. Its current researchers report that if you were to "take all eighty-four years of the Harvard Study and boil it down to a single principle for living, one life investment that is supported by similar findings across a variety of studies, it would be this: *Good relationships keep us healthier and happier. Period*" (Waldinger & Schulz, 2023, p. 10). This means you can take charge of and maximize your health and well-being by prioritizing relationships. The healthiest people at age 80 report having the greatest relationship satisfaction in their 50s (Waldinger, 2015). In line with this thinking, IFS health therapy emphasizes the relational nature of healing at every level.

One explanation for the large effect of relationships on health is that relational safety moves our brains and bodies into a "physiological state of healing that primes us to recuperate from just about every physical and mental ailment better and faster" (Porges & Porges, 2023, p. xix). In IFS health therapy, we attend to relational safety from the beginning. As parts stop being afraid and ashamed during treatment, the client's external relationships come into focus. As parts have the opportunity to heal their relational injuries with the assistance of the Self, clients naturally start to seek more balanced, satisfying external relationships. They know intuitively what research tells us: Social support and positive external relationships are crucial for physical as well as emotional well-being. Accordingly, treatment should include information about options for group and community support.

The Therapeutic Relationship in IFS

IFS health therapy attends to the client's relationships in the following ways:

1. The therapeutic relationship
2. Internal relationships between protective parts and the Self
3. Internal relationships between vulnerable parts and the Self
4. The relationship of the body and various symptoms to parts
5. External relationships with supportive individuals and groups

Importantly, the healing process is held by the IFS therapeutic relationship. Rather than being a destination, relational healing is a permanent Self-to-parts commitment (*I will be available; I will listen; I will act on your behalf*) to a compassionate process. In IFS, we assume that feelings are not shameful or dangerous, everything can be discussed, and conflict can be resolved. Additionally, the therapeutic relationship in IFS starts from the premise that we *all* have parts. That means old relational and identity wounds can always resurface in the context of the therapeutic relationship, and they generally do. This phenomenon, which Freud dubbed *transference* and *countertransference*, is an opportunity for healing. From an IFS perspective, transference signals the presence of a part who is confusing the past with the present. Countertransference is the same phenomenon, but in the therapist. Transference and countertransference tell us that (1) a part is blended, (2) this part is stuck in the past and will repeat relational patterns from the past, and (3) the part is showing or telling its story. Our goal is to help the part unblend so the client's (or therapist's) Self can update it and kindly intervene with the cycle of repetition.

We assume that any negative beliefs, feelings, and behaviors signal burdened parts. However, we also assume that these protectors are doing their jobs from a sense of necessity. We believe in their inherent goodness. We know the client will be kind and compassionate if their parts unblend. We meet their parts with curiosity about the mind-body and ask, "How are you are trying to help?"

While we expect clients' parts to blend regularly, we may be more easily taken off guard when one of *our* own reactive parts blends. Accordingly, it's our job to know our internal system and to notice when a part takes hold physically, emotionally, cognitively, or behaviorally. Our priority is the *client's* health and healing. We commit to noticing, unblending from, and helping our parts if they react to a client's part. Everything that needs to be talked about in service to the client's healing is on the table. Your unblending challenge is to notice your parts while also noticing the clients' parts. You may choose to speak for your parts—aiming for not too much or too little—or not.

The Power Differential

Our professional role endows us with power and authority in the therapeutic relationship—most blatantly, we have the power to label, pathologize, and hospitalize. It also assigns us responsibilities, including to be mindful of this power differential and to remain attuned to the client's needs. However, our ability to see clearly will always be occluded when parts blend. Other people can usually see our blind spots before we can, and as therapists we are no exception. We owe our clients a big dose of humility.

When one of our parts affects a client negatively, we can reconnect and repair by going through the usual steps of IFS with that part and being aware of our own shame cycle (Sweezy, 2023). We must ask ourselves: "Is my critical team working overtime? Are my young parts activated? Are my firefighters ramping up to distract or soothe?" We must have good relationships with all our parts: (1) our perfectionistic inner critics, (2) our vulnerable exiles who have felt shameful, and (3) our reactive firefighters. We must be able to maintain the Self's bird's-eye perspective even when our parts activate in response to a client. Reactivity is always an opportunity for professional, personal, and spiritual healing and growth.

Of course, we make mistakes sometimes; therapists have to be good enough, not perfect. In IFS, the goal is *compassionate imperfection*:

- Having openhearted, inclusive compassion for the human condition
- Caring sincerely for our clients and striving to do no harm
- Noticing our own defensive or otherwise invalidating parts
- Making repairs if our parts cause the client distress

This last component of shameless imperfection—repairing the therapeutic relationship when our parts have caused distress—is what we'll talk about next.

Self-Led Repair

When clients experience us as disconnected, unattuned, disinterested, slighting, shaming, judgmental, or domineering, they will communicate their feelings, either subtly and implicitly or clearly and directly. For example, they may:

- Say they are upset
- Sigh or huff during an exhale
- Change their body language or posture
- Turn or look away
- Fall silent or become less responsive
- Look bored, annoyed, or tense
- Glance at the clock
- Seem physically uncomfortable or fidgety
- Avoid eye contact
- Cancel appointments, come late, or not show up

If you see signs of distress in response to something you've said or done, find out what happened and do an attuned, Self-led repair. Be curious about the affected parts and express your openhearted compassion. If your parts also get scared, do a quick internal check to reassure them that you can handle the situation. The client needs your attention and attunement. Depending on the situation and the client's parts, repair can include one or all of the following steps (not necessarily in this order). Any one step may be sufficient. Ask what the client needs and wants.

1. **Acknowledge the situation:** If you see something, say something. Many clients have had the experience of being invisible and feeling unseen. When you notice discomfort, ask what's going on (unless you believe that's not what the client needs at this moment). Describe what you see in neutral language: "You seem quieter than usual this morning, and you canceled our last appointment. What's going on?"

2. **Offer compassion and care:** Don't avoid or try to fix the client's distress; be attuned and Self-led. If this is a challenge for your parts, ask them to sit next to you or go to a comfortable spot elsewhere. Then let the client know you care about their well-being: "If I've said or done something that upsets you, I want to know. Your feelings matter to me."

3. **Speak for your parts:** As you listen or reflect on a moment of disconnection, be aware of your parts. Are they giving you space? Hear their intentions and point out their impact. If it's the right call, speak for them from Self: "An excited part came up for me just now. It was sure that thought would be helpful, but I can see it wasn't. I interrupted you."

4. **Validate the client's feelings:** As you reflect on the moment of disconnection, tune in to your parts and identify what you can share that will validate the client's perceptions and feelings, using the client's language to describe them: "I can see why you felt alone and angry when my excited part came up and took over just now. I was not in touch with you."

5. **Apologize:** Model being with the client's human experience without having to determine what's right and wrong. Name your behavior and state your intention: "I'm sorry that I wasn't aware of my part and how it affected you. My job is to be here for you."

6. **Go forward with Self-leadership:** Externally, stay curious, keep acknowledging the client's experience and feelings, get permission to check in with their parts, and see what's needed. Internally, do a U-turn. Help your protective parts detach from the idea that they should be able to control the outcome of this interaction. Validate their good intentions, ask what made them reactive, offer to help the exile they protect, and get their permission before going to the exile.

This repair process invites the client to practice being assertive about their needs and models a way to be graceful and thoughtful about taking responsibility for relational transgressions. You get the opportunity to (1) communicate that you trust the client, (2) suggest a mutual agreement that both of you will speak for your parts should something feel off, and (3) illustrate what it means to speak for your parts and offer a Self-led repair. Misattunement, misunderstandings, and disagreements that affect the therapeutic relationship are all opportunities to practice the skill of Self-led, relational communication.

General Guidelines for a Self-Led Repair

- Slow down and listen.
- Be brief when you speak.
- Take care of any of your parts who feel uncomfortable.
- Leave time and space for the client to respond.
- Reassure your parts that silence is okay.
- If you think the interaction is complete, ask the client if they feel the same way. If not, do they want to keep going now or return to the discussion another time?

In addition, a Self-led repair asserts our faith in the inherent goodness and worthiness of parts and shows the client how to have challenging conversations without blaming and shaming. Self-led repairs promote a secure therapeutic relationship, which both models respectful, nonexploitive behavior and supports the client's Self as the internal source of stability and healing for the self-inflicted wound of internal shaming. As clients feel emboldened by the experience of Self-energy, some opt for fewer, closer relationships, while others expand their relational universe.

Parts and the Chronic Stress Cycle

In order for us and our clients to get to know and trust each other, we must identify which protectors are relevant to the client's illness and offer them a hopeful path forward, which includes addressing their concerns and fears. We can't liberate protectors from their chronic stress or extreme behaviors without helping the parts they protect. They need compassion and guidance, but they have to be willing to accept it.

Accordingly, the majority of treatment time goes to both the therapist and the client forming solid Self-to-protectors relationships. In particular, we identify the parts associated with illness and prioritize protectors who affect the client's health, like Tina's firefighter who soothed her exiles with dissociative late-night snacking and TV watching. To do so, we use the *chronic stress cycle* (illustrated in the following handout) to explore the biological, psychological, and social roots of the client's health problems.

Each of the points in the chronic stress cycle described here can influence or be influenced by the other points:

1. **Intense or chronic external stress:** This occurs as a result of contact with stressful or traumatic social, institutional, family, political, or physical environments. The conditions of the settings where we grow up, work, live, and grow old are known as the *social determinants of health*.

2. **Chronic internal stress:** Clients internalize stress due to legacy burdens that derive from their family, cultural, or social history, including large-scale events (e.g., war, poverty, terrorism) and personal burdens from either adult or childhood trauma and unmet developmental needs.

3. **Persistent autonomic nervous system stress response states:** The client enters a state of fight or flight, freeze/shutdown, or fawn or appease. Additionally, ongoing fear, anxiety, and stress can lead to dysregulation of the HPA axis.

4. **Emotional and physiological dysregulation:** Chronic stress can lead to overworked physiological systems and result in negative health consequences (recall *allostatic load* from chapter 2) and emotional dysregulation.

5. **Polarization between protectors in extreme roles:** Parts in extreme roles double down on opposing coping strategies. This escalating cycle of inhibition and disinhibition interrupts eating, sleep, and activity levels; exacerbates addictive behaviors; and generally leads to more stress.

6. **Negative effects of a dysregulated internal system on work and social relationships:** Clients may experience symptoms of depression (e.g., irritability, fatigue, rumination, isolation, loneliness) or anxiety (e.g., worry, avoidance, reassurance-seeking).

7. **Epigenetic modifications:** Extreme coping strategies for chronic stress raise the risk of epigenetic modifications, increasing the likelihood that a genetic predisposition for disease will be expressed. Chronic stress, cortisol exposure, and inflammation can lead to shortened telomeres, which are the protective caps on the ends of chromosomes. Telomere erosion is associated with an increased risk of degenerative diseases and cancer (Chakravarti et al., 2021; Lin & Epel, 2022).

8. **Chronic stress–related problems:** Lacking support, these parts bear the stress of diseases, syndromes, and illnesses alone inside and out, further taxing the body.

The Chronic Stress Cycle*

8. Chronic Stress–Related Problems
Heroic parts bear the stress of illness and disease

1. Intense or Chronic External Stress
Dysregulated external systems:
- Environments
- Institutions
- People

2. Chronic Internal Stress
- Toxic stress; burdens of fear
- Shame, trauma, unmet needs
- Legacy burdens

3. Persistent Autonomic Nervous System Response States
- Fight or flight
- Freeze (shutdown)
- Fawn
- Appease
- Chronic stress hormones

4. Emotional and Physiological Dysregulation
- Extreme emotional response; self-harm
- Allostatic overload: immune, gut, neuroendocrine, cardiometabolic

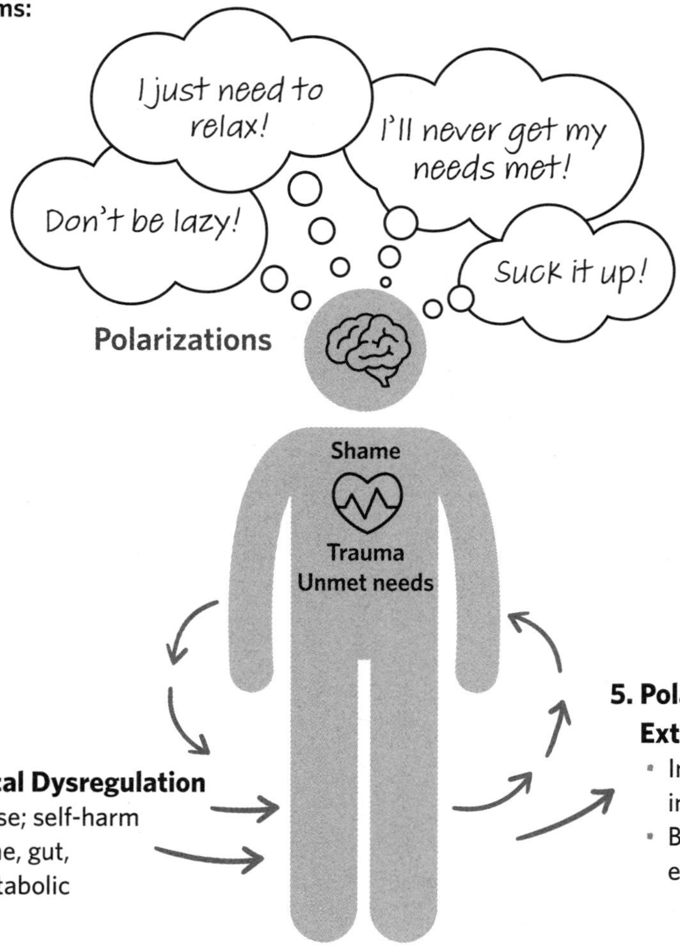

5. Polarization Between Protectors in Extreme Roles
- Increasing polarization: repressive inhibition vs. reactive rebellion
- Behaviors and addictions affect sleep, eating, physical activity, life balance

6. Negative Effects of a Dysregulated Internal System on Work and Social Relationships
- Fight or flight, fawn or appease
- Mood swings and irritability
- Anxiety, heightened threat perception
- Fatigue, depression, isolation

7. Epigenetic Modifications
- Change in gene expression
- Stress and behavioral influence on genetic predisposition
- Chronic stress leads to telomere erosion

* Adapted from Sowell (2023).

To understand how the chronic stress cycle looks in practice, recall Tina from chapter 2, who came to IFS health therapy hoping to improve her recently diagnosed metabolic syndrome to avoid type 2 diabetes and cardiovascular disease. In the following dialogue, Tina and her therapist begin to flesh out the relationships among her parts and index each issue to the appropriate point on the chronic stress cycle. We have bolded Tina's statements to highlight the thoughts, feelings, and behaviors of parts that are being identified as the session begins:

THERAPIST: When we talked about the pandemic, you described different parts that use different coping strategies for stress.

TINA: Yes, I said **I'm a fixer, not a feeler**.

THERAPIST: Yes. Fixing is an important strategy.

TINA: For me, it's a big one. I also said how **awful I feel about gaining weight by watching TV and snacking after the kids are in bed.** You explained that those parts are trying to help me.

THERAPIST: That's right. You noticed that one part eats to feel better when you're exhausted, while another worries about you getting diabetes or heart disease.

TINA: Yes. I've been thinking about that a lot.

Point 1: Chronic external stress from the pandemic

Point 2: Chronic stress from the over-responsibility of fixing and avoiding feelings, weight shame, and the fear of developing diabetes and heart disease

Point 3: Autonomic dysregulation from ongoing fight-or-flight responses during the pandemic, countered by evening shutdown and dissociation

Point 4: Allostatic load and metabolic syndrome related to coping behaviors and their consequences: nightly eating and dissociation in front of the TV, increased food cravings and intake, and a sense of responsibility to "fix" things

Point 5: The stress of polarized protectors with opposite coping strategies: eating vs. worrying, shaming and criticizing vs. trying to control

THERAPIST: How has this perspective been sitting with you?

TINA: It makes sense. **I do comfort-eat, criticize myself, and worry**. That is me—they are me.

Tina tries new language.

THERAPIST: Right. They are you—but not all of you. Want to learn more about these parts?

TINA: I'm up for it. Especially if it will help keep my blood sugar and cholesterol from getting worse.

Tina was becoming aware that her behaviors (e.g., comfort-eating), thoughts (e.g., worries and self-criticism), and feelings of shame were coming from parts. Using handouts like *The Chronic Stress Cycle* and *Signs and Symptoms of Allostatic Load* can help clients understand the mind-body connections between the stress they experience, burdened parts, and disease. The following descriptions highlight these connections for Tina:

1. **Chronic stress,** like the pandemic, combined with the internal stress of parts in extreme roles (e.g., fixers, shaming critics, shamed exiles, rebels) can keep the long-term stress response (HPA axis) active, leading to the persistent release of cortisol, a primary stress hormone.
2. **Prolonged high cortisol** levels promote the storage of visceral fat in the abdomen around the internal organs, which actively releases hormones and inflammatory substances that disrupt the balance of the metabolic and hormonal systems, promoting inflammation.
3. **Visceral fat** can increase resistance to leptin, a hormone that prompts the feeling of fullness, which can cause an increase in appetite even when we've eaten enough to meet our body's needs.
4. **Metabolic changes** from chronic stress and visceral fat lead to increased insulin resistance, elevated triglycerides, higher levels of LDL (bad) cholesterol levels, and lower levels of HDL (good) cholesterol.
5. **The inflammatory response** triggered by persistent cortisol exposure, along with the proinflammatory substances (cytokines) secreted by visceral fat, can activate immune cells and promote chronic, low-grade systemic inflammation linked to chronic inflammatory diseases, like type 2 diabetes and cardiovascular diseases.

When parts feel safe and understood, they have less stress and fear, which always feels better. Tina was blaming herself for the weight gain and metabolic syndrome without awareness of parts, but she also wasn't aware that there were physiological mechanisms in play. Tina was relieved to learn that her *cardiometabolic* disruptions like insulin resistance and high blood pressure—so named because of their effect on the cardiovascular and metabolic systems—were influenced by chronic stress and the interplay of physiological changes and the behavior of her parts. Tina was caught in a vicious cycle of chronic stress that influenced her metabolism and hormonal system, affecting her eating, sleep, and lack of activity as she sought escape through TV. With support and changes in the internal family system, the cycle can be altered.

To illustrate how this process can look with a different set of health concerns, let us introduce you to Ronan, a white man in his early 50s who identifies as a recovering alcoholic. He has a history of physical abuse by an alcoholic father (who abandoned the family when Ronan was five) and an older boy in the neighborhood. His mother worked long hours for low pay and struggled financially as a single parent. Early on, Ronan had young protectors who acted tough during and after school. Nonetheless, an older boy in the neighborhood bullied him every day, often choking him until he passed out. In turn, he struggled to focus, follow instructions, sit still, and resist the urge to speak out of turn or move about compulsively. When he was predictably labeled a "bad kid," his parts believed it. In therapy, his initial description of these years was factual and sadly sardonic: "I always got in trouble at school. Luckily, I was good at something. I could run."

When Ronan began IFS health therapy, he was a hard-driving owner of a commercial landscaping company with a host of medical problems, including headaches, neck and back pain, digestive problems, high blood pressure, and sleep disturbance. He came to therapy asking for help with his medical problems, which he believed his intense anger was making worse. He described himself as a hardworking, tense, easily angered guy with high standards and extreme reactions to stress at work. He arrived at his first session with a headache and spoke angrily about the day's events. In the dialogue that follows, we have bolded certain statements to indicate the presence of four different parts: (1) an angry, reactive part, (2) a polarized critical part who wanted to stop this reactivity but couldn't, (3) a part who felt ashamed, and (4) a shaming part. We have also indicated where these identified parts show up on the chronic stress cycle.

RONAN: **I went off on some of the guys at work again!** [*angry part*] I saw the explosion coming, but **couldn't stop it** [*critical part*]. These two young guys who work for me are fucking careless and don't think ahead! They make mistakes that cost money and time on a job that's already over budget! I cursed them out and slammed my boot into a massive tool caddy like a lunatic!

> **Point 1:** Chronic external stress due to intense work pressures
>
> **Point 2:** Chronic internal stress due to feeling shameful
>
> **Point 3:** Autonomic dysregulation of the fight response
>
> **Point 4:** Emotional and physiological dysregulation and allostatic load
>
> **Point 5:** Parts driven into extreme roles by the dysregulation of the fight response
>
> **Point 6:** Negative impacts on work and relationships

THERAPIST: How are you feeling in your body as you remember this?

RONAN: Right now, my neck and back are like a rock, and my stomach is churning.* I feel **like an ass** [*ashamed part*]. I've always done this. Why can't I control myself? I'm **an immature idiot!** [*shaming part*]

> **Point 2:** Chronic internal stress due to fear, shamefulness, and unmet needs
>
> **Point 4:** Emotional dysregulation due to physiological dysregulation from at-the-ready rage, seen in muscle tension and digestive problems
>
> **Point 5:** A protective part shaming and an exile feeling shameful

THERAPIST: This isn't your fault, Ronan. It's—

RONAN: [*Interrupting*] Oh, come on! Of course it's my fault!

> A manager part speaks.

THERAPIST: It is certainly your responsibility, but otherwise we'll have to agree to disagree because I'm confident it's not your fault.

> The therapist is a hope merchant.

RONAN: [*Condescending and skeptical, yet curious*] You're going to say it's a part, right?

---

* While we know that these physical symptoms Ronan describes are related to tension and stress from one or more parts, more information is needed to determine whether these symptoms are related to a single part or multiple parts.

Therapist: Yes, one who is reacting to your nervous system under stress. We may find that some of your physical symptoms are also related to stress.

Ronan: Say what? I go off on those guys, act like an ass, make myself sick with headaches, stomach problems, and high blood pressure. But it's all . . . *Oh, it's just my nervous system. I'm not responsible!* I don't want permission to go on being a jerk.

> This manager part fears Ronan's firefighter parts will get off the hook.

Therapist: Stress affects your body. I'm guessing your nervous system is in a chronic state of fight or flight and needs help. Why? Well, your past can go on being a source of stress in the present. It may sound strange to you, but I can help you help your body by getting in relationship with your parts.

Ronan: It does sound strange.

Therapist: When we feel threatened, the body releases stress hormones like adrenaline and cortisol, which change how we think and feel in preparation for fighting or fleeing. Threat tends to activate our parts who feel most powerless. You can notice and decide if this is true for you.

Ronan: Okay. So, let's say my automatic reactions are not my fault and I'm not in charge, which I don't believe. Are you saying I can't do anything about it?

> Ronan has no concept of resources beyond his polarized protectors.

Therapist: You can do a lot about it! Can I show you? Are you up for that?

> Offering hope and a chance to check it out, the therapist gets permission to proceed.

Ronan: I am!

> The client's protectors signal a preliminary willingness to try something new.

Therapist: Okay. We'll start by finding out how your parts react to danger signals from your nervous system.

As this dialogue illustrates, Ronan's physical symptoms were a result of the wear and tear his mind-body had endured from being in a chronic fight-or-flight response:

1. **Anger:** The mind's focus becomes narrow and external; muscles tense up in the legs, torso, shoulders, neck, and jaw; the hands may go into fists; the heart beats faster; and blood flows away from extremities like the fingers and toes to large muscles like the thighs, heart, and biceps.
2. **Headaches, neck, and back pain:** The stress response contracts the muscles, especially in the shoulders, neck, and upper back, in preparation for defense. With chronic stress, these muscles stay partially contracted, which is painful and can lead to reduced blood and oxygen flow, as well as impaired waste removal, resulting in more aching and fatigue. Additionally, stress can contribute to inflammation, increased pain sensitivity, and poor sleep—all of which can exacerbate pain.

3. **Digestive problems:** Since the fight-or-flight response prioritizes blood flow to vital organs, such as the heart and muscles, and simultaneously decreases blood flow for nonessential functions, including digestion, this can lead to nausea, indigestion, or changes in bowel function.

4. **High blood pressure:** Stress hormones constrict blood vessels, raising blood pressure. If the threat passes, this physiological response subsides. But for people like Ronan, who feel endangered and remain on high alert all the time, it may not.

5. **Sleep disturbance:** The feeling of being in constant danger—and the fight-or-flight activation that goes with that feeling—can disrupt sleep at onset or later in the night.

Ronan and Tina illustrate what it's like to live in the present in a body that is being affected by parts who are trapped in the past. For exiled parts and their dedicated protectors, the past is not over. They continue to experience past events, and current stressors allow them to send a message: *This happened before and it's not over yet for me.* Protectors understand this but don't know how to help.

Engaging with Parts

Like Tina and Ronan, many clients don't arrive at IFS health therapy talking about fear and emotional dysregulation or a history of trauma because their protective parts are successfully hiding these vulnerabilities. Instead, they talk about their health problems and, sometimes, current stressors. (We call these topics *trailheads* because by inquiring in that direction, the client will find parts who need help.) At the same time, their body tells a story. For example, it wasn't until later in treatment, when Tina began listening inside and got to know her parts, that she became aware that the metabolic syndrome conditions she was diagnosed with (e.g., insulin resistance, hypertension, high cholesterol) were linked to her experiences of immigration trauma, loss, and chronic internal stress. But, as we saw in her early sessions, she was very aware of (1) pandemic stressors, (2) the cost of stress eating, and (3) the possibility of developing type 2 diabetes or heart disease. At this point, she spoke *from* (not *for*) shaming parts who were frantic about her weight and the stress eating. Many clients who have health problems present in this way. Shaming, critical parts are a great place to start because they want to be heard, they need to be reassured, and shaming actually drives the disinhibited behavior (in Tina's case, eating) they wish to inhibit.

Ronan also described being aware of (1) external stressors at work, (2) physical symptoms (in his case, related to the chronic dysregulation that followed from an ongoing fight-or-flight response), (3) shaming self-judgment, (4) subsequent feelings of shamefulness, and (5) rageful reactivity toward others that affected his relationships and exacerbated his shame and chronic stress. But it wasn't until he listened to his protectors that he discovered that the different coping strategies causing him so much internal stress were driven by the shame, trauma, and unmet childhood needs of the boy inside—who had been abandoned, terrorized by a violent bully, and shamed in school for his difficulty focusing. That boy had come to believe *he* was the problem. His banishment to the unconscious by his protectors reinforced his belief.

Tina and Ronan both had some conscious awareness of their parts and did not object to the IFS therapist using parts language. This helps clients notice their parts and encourages the parts to unblend—a major goal of treatment. Not all clients take as readily to the concept of parts or to IFS vernacular. Objections don't have to be a barrier to IFS treatment, but they require flexibility and patience.

Although Tina and Ronan were vaguely aware of and not startled by the concept of parts, neither of them had perspective on their parts. Their parts were still doing the talking, and Tina and Ronan were not yet listening and thinking, *Hmm. This sounds like a part.* That is the next step, where we support the client to drop into their mind-body and engage their parts. We do so by noticing some characteristic of a part on the chronic stress cycle and expand from there. For example, we might notice:

- A behavior (e.g., Tina's stress eating; Ronan's yelling at his employees)
- A strong emotion (e.g., Tina's anxiety; Ronan's rage)
- A state of being (e.g., Tina's exhaustion; Ronan's churning stomach, headaches, and muscle tension)
- A momentary somatic, emotional, or behavioral mind-body experience (e.g., Tina's onset of dread; Ronan's urge to kick the tool caddy)

To notice the part more fully, we ask questions:

- "Do any thoughts or feelings go with that [*e.g., physical sensation, behavior, desire*]?"
- "Do any behavioral urges go with the part's [*e.g., pain, thought, emotion, sensation*]?"

These questions nudge the client to get curious about their parts. As their parts, in turn, become increasingly aware of the client's Self, they share more about their ongoing emotional distress, physiological dysregulation, and toxic identity beliefs. By turning our attention to stress in the body and parts who are willing to speak (or otherwise communicate), we discover who has been affected by chronic stress.

For example, engaging with parts allowed us to discover that Tina has a set of anxious managers who are intensely active and productive during the day, and a team of firefighters that activates at night, escaping into TV and dissociative comfort-eating. Similarly, Ronan has a reproving manager who is intensely critical of him all the time, a rageful firefighter who lashes out at others, and a ruminating, obsessional manager who focuses in the evening on his success and reputation in business. In short, despite their different presentations, both Tina and Ronan display signs of emotional and physiological dysregulation; both have shaming, critical parts as well as parts who feel shameful; and both report increasing awareness and understanding of their behaviors when they feel less stressed. At the same time, they are both mired in the ineffective, costly coping strategies (e.g., overwork, high performance standards, harsh criticism) of some underpowered, frightened protectors.

When mounting external stressors touch on Ronan's identity and trauma burdens, he becomes rageful. In turn, his emotional and physiological dysregulation affect his sleep, digestion, anxiety level, physical pain, and more. When mistakes and mishaps occur at work, he feels inadequate and fears criticism. His rageful firefighter part comes to the rescue by blaming his employees, which harms those relationships and activates his critical manager team. As they take his disinhibited, angry part to task, Ronan's body and all his other parts take another trip around the chronic stress cycle.

To avoid aggravating the client's emotional and physical state during treatment, we start by focusing on a protector, often a manager who is concerned about the extreme behavior of some other part (like Ronan's critical part who fears his rageful part). In the dialogue that follows, Ronan engages two of his parts to learn how they respond to emotional and physiological dysregulation and how their different responses put them at odds.

THERAPIST: It sounds like your rageful part stirs up strong reactions in you and other people.

RONAN: Yeah, it sure does. I'm very critical of myself. I'm a conscientious person. I've been clean and sober for a long time. I don't respect raging. I want to be in control, which sounds strange since I can be so out of control!

This illustrates a polarization between two of Ronan's protective parts, who have opposing survival strategies.

THERAPIST: So, there's a highly reactive part who rages. [*Ronan nods.*] And there's a highly conscientious part who wants to keep things under control. [*He nods again.*] What a tough combination!

Confirming understanding with the client and mapping it out

RONAN: Yeah, that's me, from one extreme to the other. I'm either very controlled or very uncontrolled. And when I'm out of control, I just can't stop. I want to, but it would be like slamming on the brakes while driving 100 miles an hour. That's how it feels to me.

THERAPIST: That's a great description of a physical state. A surge of adrenaline causes an immediate, intense fight-or-flight response in your body.

RONAN: I never thought of it as physical. I just call myself an asshole. Sorry!

THERAPIST: No need to apologize. I've heard the word before. But let's think who might warm up and be more cooperative with an apology.

RONAN: Who?

THERAPIST: One of your parts is insulting another part. Let's start there.

RONAN: Oh! We're talking parts?! Okay, I have a part who's an asshole. For sure. I'm not going to apologize for telling the truth.

The critical part reacts negatively.

THERAPIST: Are you open to hearing my perspective on what's happening inside you right now? [*Ronan nods.*] You are seeing things through the eyes of the critical part. Its perspective is important and legitimate, but incomplete. Would it—and you—be willing to hear directly from the angry part about why it explodes?

Validating a part polarized with another and asking for cooperation.

RONAN: Maybe . . . Do you judge me for being angry?

The critical part fears Ronan will be judged for getting angry.

THERAPIST: Angry parts have important messages for us. I'd like to hear from yours. Beyond that, I assume that both the critical and the angry part want you to be the best version of yourself. They're each trying to help you, but it's not going well and we can help them.

RONAN: [*After a pause*] That's true. [*Choking up*] They do want the "best me" and it's not going well. But the critical part wants to talk first.

THERAPIST: How do you feel toward the critical part?

RONAN: I want to hear him, I guess. But, you know, I feel like that *is* me.

> This is the first time Ronan has referred to the critic as *him*.

THERAPIST: I know. And he is really you, but just one *part* of you. What does he want you to know?

> The therapist switches now to the same gendered pronoun.

RONAN: He just, you know, really dislikes that raging part, all right?

Shifting to Explicit Direct Access When a Protector Won't Unblend

We say a part is *blended* when it has taken over internally. This is what happened in the preceding dialogue—Ronan was blended with the critical part. This critical part would try to shame Ronan's rageful part into silence and submission, but when this caused Ronan's vulnerable parts to feel ashamed, the rageful part would take over anyway. We call the critic's combative relationship with the rageful part a *protector polarization*. As Ronan's critical and rageful parts squared off, they became more extreme. Entrenched internal conflicts like this are very stressful and hard on the body.

When the therapist suggested getting to know the angry part, the critical part (who was afraid of Ronan getting close to the rageful one) said he wanted to be heard first. Since Ronan was far more comfortable with his critic, this was a good idea. In fact, Ronan was so identified (blended) with the critic that the therapist decided at the outset of their chat to talk with it directly. Remember, this is called *explicit direct access*, which means the therapist's Self temporarily takes the lead and, while referring to the client in the third person, asks questions about the part's relationship with the client (e.g., "What do you do for Ronan?"). In addition to being an efficient way of getting to know a part who won't unblend, direct access helps the client (1) *notice* the blended part, (2) *listen* as it speaks, and (3) *learn* about it.

During explicit direct access, you ask questions that help the client learn more about how their physical symptoms relate to a blended part, how it's trying to help, who it protects, and what it fears:

1. To begin, ask the client how they notice the part. They might say physically, emotionally, or in their thoughts, beliefs, or actions.

2. Next, ask the client's whole internal system to let this part blend fully, with no pushback from other parts, as well as no thinking or censorship. Invite them all to listen as this part answers your questions.

3. Now ask this part some questions:
   - "What do you do for [*client's name*]?"
   - "What's the worst thing that would happen if you stopped doing this job?"
   - "What effect do you have on the body?"
   - "What worries you most?"
   - "Who do you protect?"
     - If it protects another part, ask:
       - "What if [*client's name*] could help that part feel better and keep it safe?"
     - If it protects another person, ask:
       - "What would happen to [*client's name*] if you stopped taking care of them?"
       - "What happens to [*client's name*] when you prioritize taking care of this other person?"
       - "If [*client's name*] could get you out of being responsible for this other person, would you be interested?"
   - "What do you need from [*client's name*]?"
4. Tell the part you're going to talk with the client again, and then ask the client: "What is it like to listen to this part? How do you feel toward the part now? What would you like to say to the part after hearing about its motives and concerns?"

Although proactive managers want healthy functioning, when they become extreme and polarize with reactive firefighters who seek immediate relief from stress, our job (collectively, therapist and client) is to recognize the validity of both needs and not banish either side. Attention is a powerful tool. Once Ronan noticed the blended critic, it caused the critic, in turn, to notice Ronan, which is the first step toward our goal of separation or *unblending*. In this case, the therapist had to convince two parts—the critic and the angry part—not to blend. Children who grow up in dysregulated external systems, as Ronan did, have no choices and no power. Ronan had reason to be angry, but being angry put him at greater risk. Accordingly, his critic was constantly trying to suppress his anger. In the following dialogue, the therapist uses explicit direct access to engage Ronan's blended, active, dominant critic.

Therapist: Ronan, would you like to invite the critical part who dislikes the raging to blend with you? I'll talk to him while you listen. [*Ronan nods and closes his eyes.*] Let me know when you feel the part fully.

Ronan: [*After a pause*] Yes. Now.

Therapist: Notice the physical aspects of this conscientious you.

Directing Ronan to notice how this part shows up, somatically or otherwise

Ronan: My neck and shoulders feel like rock. It's uncomfortable.

Therapist: How often do you feel this way?

Ronan: Most of the time. The back of my head, neck, and shoulders is almost always tense.

Therapist: What thoughts and feelings go with this tension?

Ronan: [*Pauses.*] I think about the crew at work and my never-ending to-do list. I do it all the time. I keep things running smoothly. Even now I'm thinking about all the things I have to do.

Therapist: What are you concerned would happen if you didn't think about Ronan's responsibilities all the time?

> This standard question evokes the protector's fears.

Ronan: Things wouldn't work out. He'd drop the ball and everything would fall apart. That raging part would take over or something else would go wrong. He would fail.

Therapist: What happens if Ronan fails?

> Using a what-if question to identify the part's biggest fear

Ronan: He'd be worthless. He'd get rejected and be alone. He'd feel like he doesn't deserve to be alive.

Therapist: High stakes! That would be awful. You have powerful reasons to keep things under control.

> Validating and affirming the part

Ronan: Yeah, but it's impossible. I'm on guard all the time and things still go wrong. It literally hurts. [*Ronan places a hand on the back of his neck.*]

> The critic admits defeat.

Therapist: I see that! [*Pauses.*] Thank you. I'm going to talk with Ronan again, and now you can listen. [*He nods.*] Ronan, have you been listening to this conversation?

> Shifting out of explicit direct access to process what the part said

Ronan: Yeah.

Therapist: How do you feel toward the conscientious part now?

> This question reveals the client's level of Self-energy.

Ronan: Grateful.

Therapist: How did that part feel when you put your hand on his tense neck?

Ronan: [*After a long pause*] It felt like a buddy was there with him.

Therapist: That's great. You *are* a buddy for him. I'm glad he felt that.

When Ronan placed his hand on his neck, the therapist sensed a shift and asked Ronan how he felt toward the part now. His response ("grateful") prompted the therapist to inquire further and ask how the blended part responded to his touch, reinforcing the connection between Ronan's Self and the critical part.

The touch of Ronan's hand gave the critic a powerful relational and physical moment of support—a sensory and emotional connection that he could use as a shortcut to calm and safety in the future.

Parts Mapping

During this session, Ronan and his therapist learned about several things that were happening in his mind-body. The critical part shared its fears that the rageful part would take over, everything would fall apart, and Ronan would fail. The critic warned that this would lead to Ronan being alone, feeling worthless (i.e., an exile would blend with him), and becoming suicidal. The following diagram shows what Ronan's initial parts map looked like. A *parts map* is a tool we use to visually identify the various parts in a client's system and see relationships between them. When we map parts during a session, we capture a lot of information that we can use to maintain continuity between sessions.

Ronan's Initial Parts Map

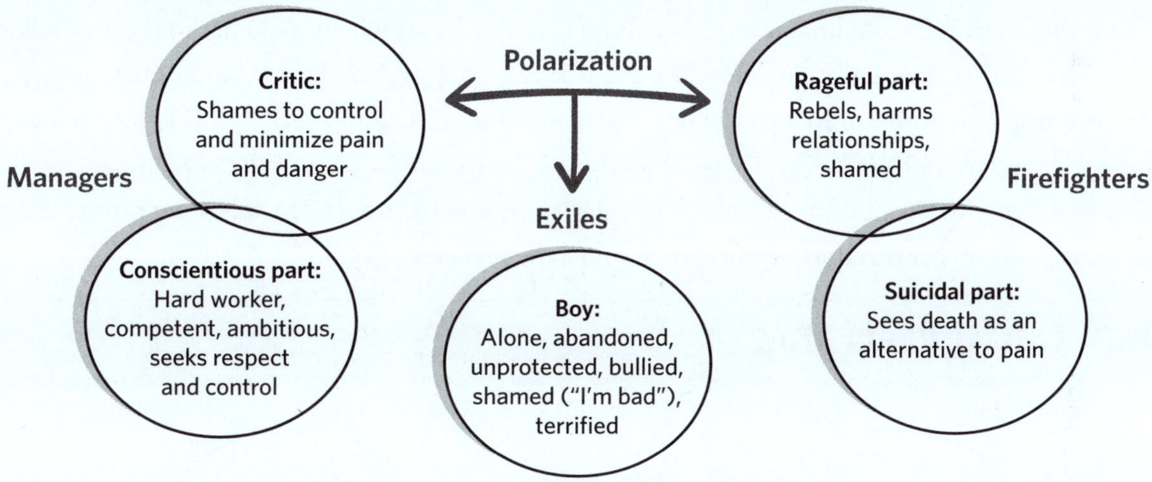

Maps are especially helpful when tracking more than one issue. We can create different parts maps of the collection of parts involved in different problems. As the client describes stressful life events and other trailheads from the past, we:

- **Jot down characteristics of the parts we're hearing about.** This can include feelings, thoughts, behaviors, reactions, physical sensations, and conflicts between parts.
- **Notice what's missing** (e.g., reactions and feelings we would expect someone to have in that situation). We ask the client to describe what they *did* feel and think, and see if there's a natural emotional response missing. We then ask if any part or feeling has been stifled. We can add these missing parts or feelings, as well as other characteristics of parts that might be missing, to the map in parentheses with a question mark to be further explored as treatment continues.
- **Use symbols to represent the relationships in client's internal system.** Typical symbols involve (1) parts, (2) polarizations between parts, (3) stress, and (4) the triangulation of polarized parts

with the exile that they protect. Parts maps can be drawn by hand spontaneously. In our example, we used circles to represent parts and paired them with descriptive words. To distinguish parts from each other, you can also draw parts in different shapes, sizes, and colors. You can use the following samples or make up your own. For example, you might choose a sun or heart for Self-energy.

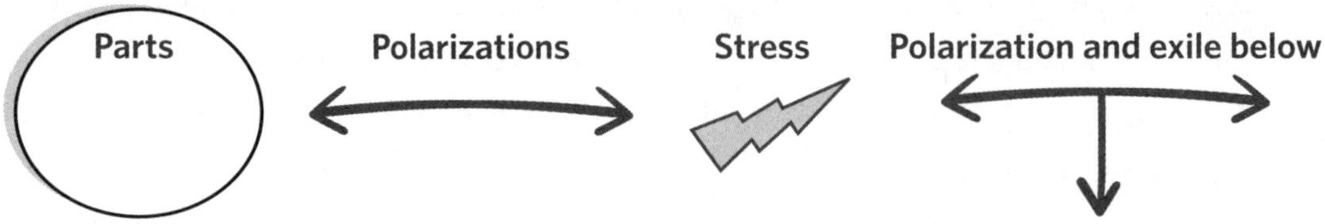

- **Place the symbols on the page in relation to each other.** Some parts will be allied and may be in close proximity or overlap. Others will be polarized and may be separated (perhaps designated by a double arrow between them). Polarized parts will have one or more exiles whom they are trying to protect in opposite ways. However, you and your client should feel free to personalize all this.

To further our discussion of parts mapping, let's return to Tina's story. Remember that in her initial assessment, she identified an internal conflict between (1) a "fixer" part who wanted her to get help following through on medical recommendations to reduce the risk of getting type 2 diabetes and cardiac disease, and (2) a stress-eating part who coped by staying up late, watching TV, and snacking. Tina also noticed the tension and disapproval of (3) a critical manager who was desperate to control the coping part, as well as (4) exiled parts who felt dread or stress from which she was trying to escape. The following provisional parts map reminds Tina and her therapist of where they ended the previous session.

Tina's Initial Parts Map

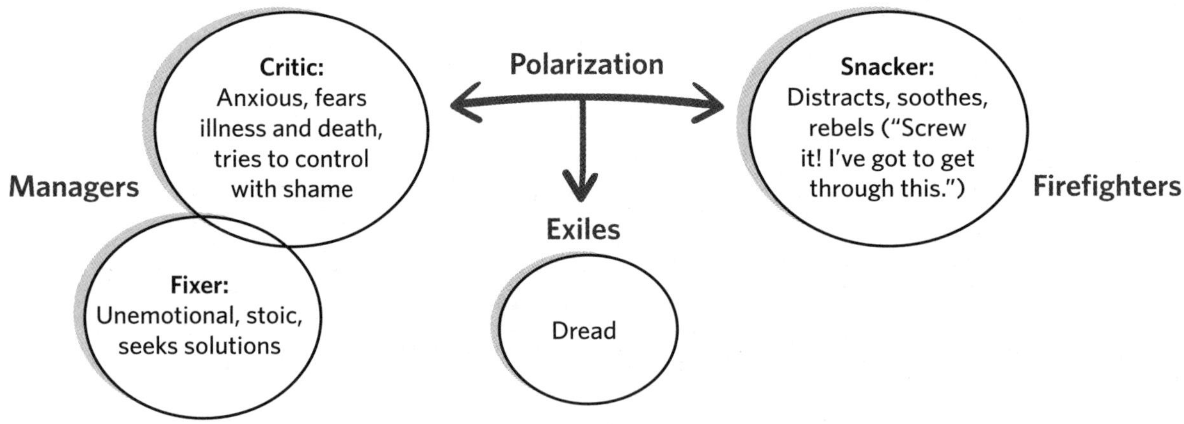

Managers keep life in order, maintain to-do lists, monitor health, and invest in therapy. Even though their socially sanctioned efforts are not controversial and seem self-evidently beneficial, unblending from them is a crucial first step in therapy. That was the focus of this next session with Tina.

Tina: What is so hard about this? When I'm not in one of those worn-down moments, I know this habit is fixable. I want to say, stop already! That's it. Just be disciplined and *stop it!*

Therapist: I noticed a change in your facial expression and how you talked about yourself just now. Did you feel that you were getting more agitated and self-critical?

Tina: I *am* agitated and mad at myself—at that part of me. I'm playing with fire. There's a simple solution, and it's so frustrating that this part of me has this habit. I just need to stop sitting around, get moving, and eat well! What is so hard?

> Tina goes between speaking *from* the manager part to speaking *about* the parts the manager finds so frustrating.

Therapist: Are you open to hearing another observation?

> Seizing the opportunity to identify polarizations

Tina: Sure.

Therapist: I hear a frustrated, critical part who is mad at "you"—which means you when you're blended with the part who distracts and soothes with late-night TV and snacks to help cope. That's the snacking part, not you. I would like both of these hardworking parts to meet you. [*Tina shakes her head.*] I believe you can help them with this dilemma.

Tina: My health dilemma?

Therapist: Yes, wanting to be healthy and feel secure while actually feeling overwhelmed and in need of relief.

Tina: You've got that right. So, what are you thinking?

Therapist: Both of these parts are trying to help, and we don't want to exile either one of them. But we do need to find a better way to solve the problem.

Tina: Right. How?

Therapist: That's the question and the crux of the matter. What I'm going to suggest may seem counterintuitive to your parts. Are they willing to keep an open mind?

Tina: I hear *maybe*.

Therapist: Okay. Maybe is fair. That's all I ask. In addition to having these hardworking, problem-solving parts, you have some more vulnerable, tender parts who have been hurt along the way in your life. They produce a lot of inner stress because they need help. There's a Tina who is *not* a part who could help them, with permission from everyone who does the protecting.

> Introducing the idea of exiles and the Self

Tina: They think that's a cute idea.

Therapist: But they're dismissing it? [*Tina nods.*] I understand. The cool thing is that they don't have to believe me to try it out. They could meet you first and decide for themselves if you are safe and if you could be useful. If they don't want your help, they don't have to take it. They're the boss.

But if they don't meet you, they'll never find out what you can do for them and also for the parts they protect.

Helping protectors feel safe by emphasizing their power

TINA: Well, you've got their interest.

THERAPIST: We're looking for a volunteer.

TINA: Okay. The critical one.

THERAPIST: Ask it to look you in the eye. Who does it see?

TINA: A weak-willed person who is getting fat and sick.

That is, the critic sees another part.

THERAPIST: Ask the part who snacks at night to separate from you and step back for a moment. It can sit right next to you. [*She nods.*] Ask the critic to look again. Who does it see now?

Asking the stress-eating part to unblend

TINA: A sad little girl.

This is now the blended part.

THERAPIST: Ask her to sit on your other side. [*She nods.*] Ask the critic to look again. Who does it see now?

Continuing to ask parts to unblend until the Self shows up

TINA: Someone it doesn't know.

This answer usually signals that the part has seen the client's Self, but we check.

THERAPIST: How's the critical part responding?

TINA: It's surprised and a bit relieved. But wary.

This answer confirms that the part has seen Tina's Self. Parts are not surprised and relieved when they see other parts.

THERAPIST: Wary?

TINA: It's saying, *Where have you been?*

This question is common when a part makes contact with Self.

THERAPIST: That's a fair question too. What do you say?

TINA: Someplace inside.

THERAPIST: Right. And you're here now. Would this critical part like your help?

TINA: Maybe.

Therapist: Maybe is a good start. Ask it to please keep speaking up and letting us know about any concerns.

Tina: Okay.

Even though Tina's protectors have gotten a glimpse of her Self, we can't predict what will happen next. They may feel reassured and relax, they may become vigilant and fearful about being replaced, or they may feel some combination of these. Regardless of what comes next, we now have a reference point for the end goal of IFS health therapy, which we call Self-leadership. Whether a little or a lot, this reference point signifies the opening of a closed door. Tina's therapist continues on through that door by bringing Tina's attention back to the current target part—the critic—and following a six-step sequence called the 6 F's to help Tina: (1) ***find*** and (2) ***focus on*** the part, (3) ask how she ***feels toward*** the part and check for access to any qualities of Self before moving on to (4) ***befriending*** the part. Once there's a relational connection with the part, the therapist can move on to (5) ***flesh out*** the part's role, its fears, and the exile it protects. The last step involves (6) addressing the ***fears*** the part has about connecting with the exiled part. (We'll talk more about the 6 F's in the next chapter.) You'll see this sequence illustrated in the following dialogue:

Therapist: Tina, how do you become aware of this worried, frustrated critic who wants to stop the snacking?

> Helping Tina *find* the part

Tina: I notice anger and frustration. I hear blame and criticism toward the snacking part.

Therapist: Do you feel the anger in your body?

> Helping Tina *focus* on the part

Tina: My shoulders get tense, my arms ache, my jaw hurts. This critical part wants to take control and force that other part to stop. I want to hit something.

Therapist: As you notice that, how do you feel toward it? [*Tina hesitates.*] Does it make sense to you, given your health risks?

> This *feel toward* question (and the following "make sense" question) check for Tina's access to the Self

Tina: Yes! It hates things feeling so out of control. It's very practical and works super hard.

Therapist: How do you feel toward the frustrated, critical part right now?

Tina: I notice that it *is* me most of the time. I get how hard it works trying to help me, like with the high blood sugar and cholesterol.

Therapist: Take your time, Tina. Let it know that you understand and appreciate its hard work.

> Helping Tina *befriend* the part

At this point, Tina's therapist quietly watches and listens for the Self's physical presence in the body. As Tina's Self embodies, her demeanor changes. Her eyes are closed, but the therapist can tell from her attentive posture and expression of interest and curiosity that she is focusing inside, not dissociating. Tina's breathing slows and deepens, her facial muscles soften, her shoulders relax and drop, her clenched jaw releases, and her whole body relaxes into the chair. The therapist follows up by checking on the Self-to-part connection.

THERAPIST: Is the critical part aware of you [*the Self*] now?

TINA: Yes. It's surprised that I'm here. But glad.

> The part's positive reception indicates that it feels connected to her Self.

THERAPIST: That's great. See what it wants you to notice or know about its role.

> Helping Tina *flesh out* the part, its role, and its purpose

TINA: [*A long pause in which she nods to herself, looking alert and calm.*]

THERAPIST: What's happening?

TINA: The critic gets that I'm listening. It's showing me what it does—how it helps me get by and succeed. It's still doing that, but it's exhausted.

> Tina's voice is full and relaxed. She's listening and attending to the part. Her positive regard and appreciation are apparent.

The therapist wants to help Tina find and connect with any exiled parts (whose feelings drive extreme protectors) as soon as possible, but pacing is key. Cooperation from the dominant critical manager—who's anxious about Tina's health and would like to control her stress-eating firefighter—is vital to progress. That part must be willing to let her proceed with the exile it protects. Therefore, the therapist must ask this question, aimed at identifying the exile: "What are you afraid would happen if you stopped doing your job?" If the manager balks at sharing this information, the therapist can explore why and address its concerns.

THERAPIST: What would happen if this critical part stopped trying to control the stress-eating part?

> *Fleshing out* this part's fears

TINA: I'd get type 2 diabetes like my mom.

THERAPIST: And if you got diabetes like your mother, what would happen to you?

> Digging deeper, looking for the fear beneath that outcome

TINA: I'd die.

THERAPIST: Is there a part who is afraid of dying? [*After a long pause, Tina suddenly opens her eyes.*] What just happened?

TINA: I saw my mother being depressed. Then the picture went away.

THERAPIST: Ask why.

TINA: I was feeling horribly sad. Then everything just stopped and got quiet.

THERAPIST: How are you feeling now?

TINA: [*Avoiding eye contact*] Spacey.

A dissociative firefighter part has stepped in

THERAPIST: Let's reorient. Let's move around. [*The therapist demonstrates and they both shift in their chairs.*] How does that feel?

TINA: [*Looking at the therapist now*] Better.

THERAPIST: What was it like to get shut down in that way?

TINA: A little frustrating, but also a relief.

THERAPIST: A relief from . . . ?

TINA: Deep sadness and maybe the dread?

THERAPIST: Okay. A protective part can take you out if it doesn't like what's happening. Most of us have that skill. It's called dissociating.

TINA: I never thought I did that. But I guess I do.

In this dialogue, Tina acknowledged feeling deep sadness and being afraid of feeling dread. She also noticed the part who came to the rescue by dissociating, as well as the relief that followed. Through this, the therapist picked up on a polarity: One part was frustrated at the interruption, while another was relieved. The therapist continued by summarizing and checking in.

THERAPIST: So, on the one hand, when you noticed the sadness and dread, everything stopped, which brought relief. On the other hand, now you notice frustration about this interruption. Is that right?

TINA: Yes. I felt sadness and then dread when we first started, and relief when the feelings stopped. But then my part that wants to get healthy felt frustrated.

THERAPIST: All that makes sense. The sadness and dread are what we call a *trailhead*. It tells us where to explore so we can find out who inside needs help. But we want to do that exploration safely. With permission from any part who has a concern, we can arrange safe conditions.

Letting Tina know they will eventually address her critical manager's *fears*

TINA: I would like that.

THERAPIST: I appreciate the wisdom of all your parts, including the one who wants you to get healthy and the one who is pointing us toward underlying, unaddressed needs. We will remember all this. To chart a path forward, let's summarize where we are and update your parts map to include all of the parts we've noticed so far.

Before the end of this session, Tina and her therapist noted the activity of her parts during the session, including the emergence of a sad little girl. This might be an exile, but it also might be a young manager. They will have to keep going to find out, as Tina's protective parts were clearly trying to keep the feelings of dread at a bay. Tina and her therapist also added the dissociative part to her parts map. The goal when maintaining a parts map is to keep adding any new information that will be helpful to track.

Tina's Parts Map, Version 2

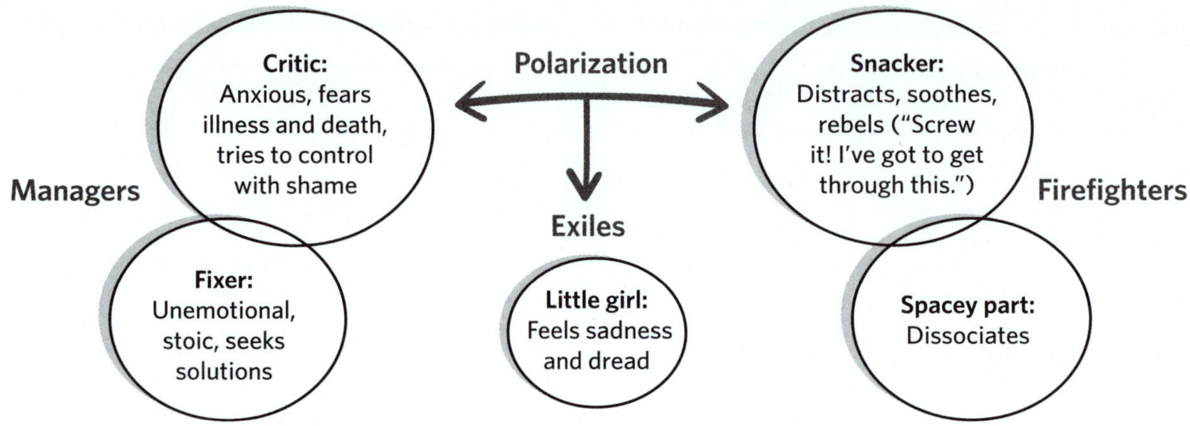

Dissociation and Parts

Dissociative parts take over when they believe the feelings, memories, or intentions of some other parts will be reminiscent of a scary, dangerous, or overwhelming time in the past. When they shut everything down inside, they are often easy to spot. Tina's dissociative protector abruptly shut down the conflict between her manager and her reactive coping part, leaving her with a sense of blankness. They can also roll in like a fog, overpower with sleepiness, or make it hard to think and articulate. Dissociative parts can also lead us to zone out—for example, by mindlessly scrolling on our screens or becoming hyper-focused on work—causing us to lose track of time as well as our inner world. A blended dissociative part may:

- Ignore the present and think about something else
- Space out
- Stare into space and avoid eye contact
- Shut down
- Forget certain places
- Forget certain people
- Forget chunks of recent time
- Forget childhood
- Sound disconnected or distracted from the moment
- Invite another part to take over abruptly and change the subject

Dissociation seems to be a hardwired capacity. Some of us have more of it than others. Protective parts use this capacity to block overwhelming or dangerous experiences that threaten to rise into awareness. These parts arise in response to reasons ranging from monotony (like driving on autopilot on a highway) to stimulation in the present that is reminiscent of an overwhelming experience in the past. Dissociative parts can disconnect us from thoughts, feelings, memories, our sense of self, our sensory and bodily awareness, our surroundings, other people, other parts, the Self, and behavioral urges. A dissociative part will use the most accessible and effective means at hand and vary its intensity to the demands of the moment.

Trauma, especially in childhood, can produce powerful dissociative parts who may not be verbal. When a person's symptoms meet the criteria for dissociative identity disorder (DID), their parts are generally disconnected from memory and each other and can be disconnected from their present environment as well. Since life is inevitably dangerous in small or big ways, and psychic protection helps, IFS health therapy thinks of dissociative parts as serving various functions, including:

- Ousting the memories, feelings, and thoughts of vulnerable, burdened parts from consciousness in favor of a focus on functioning well and carrying on with life
- Interfering with feelings, thoughts, memory, and behavior to avoid danger and maintain enough homeostasis to keep functioning
- Shaming vulnerable parts and elevating anxiety to distract from unwanted feelings, memories, and beliefs
- Engaging in repetitive self-harm to release endogenous opioids and soothe the body, or to break through the deadness of numbing by feeling physical pain

If you have little or no experience with active dissociative parts, we recommend getting supervision from a knowledgeable clinician experienced in the treatment of dissociation and dissociative parts.

Some Possible Effects of Overactive Dissociative Parts

On Self-Awareness	On Consciousness	On Perception
Feeling: • Numb • Emotionally deadened • Detached from experience • Mentally blank or distant from thoughts • Alien to one's identity or unable to recognize oneself	**Feeling:** • Unaware • Foggy • Spaced out • In a trance • Unreal (depersonalization) **Having:** • Gaps in memory • Unaccounted time • Other people describe radically different parts appearing and disappearing with no co-consciousness or awareness of each other **Engaging in:** • Robotic, purposeless behavior	**Experiencing:** • Visual distortions • Auditory distortions • Tactile distortions **Feeling:** • The world is unfamiliar or unreal (derealization) **Being unable to:** • Recognize familiar places or faces

Dissociation, Interoception, and Neuroception

Clients who seek help for an illness or a physical ailment often dissociate in response to *interoceptive signals*, which are the internal sensory signals that the organs send to the brain. Interoception is what gives us the ability to notice our internal cues, like hunger, thirst, or the need to use the bathroom, and respond accordingly. However, people who have felt trapped by another person or by chronic pain—as happens with, for example, inflammatory arthritis disease (e.g., rheumatoid arthritis, psoriatic arthritis, and ankylosing spondylitis)—often have parts who dissociate to block physical sensations and the body. At the same time, they can also have vigilant parts who are informed by *neuroception*—the neural assessment of danger and safety based on previous experience (Porges, 2022)—leading these parts to watch vigilantly for any visual, auditory, or sensory cues of environmental threat.

Interoceptive Signals

Hunger, fullness, and digestion: Hunger cues, satiety or fullness, thirst, nausea, digestive discomfort, bloating, stomach movement or emptiness, shakiness or weakness from low blood sugar

Temperature regulation: Feeling hot or warm or cold, sweating, shivering, goosebumps, flushing or warmth in the face or body

Cardiovascular sensations: Awareness of heartbeat, palpitations, pounding or fluttering, changes in rhythm or intensity, sensations associated with blood-pressure shifts (e.g., lightheadedness or pressure)

Respiratory sensations: Breathing rate (fast or slow), depth of breath (shallow or deep), breath hunger, tightness in the chest or throat, urges to sigh or yawn

Musculoskeletal sensations: Pain, tension, stiffness, relaxation or release, fatigue, internal vibrations, restlessness, body position awareness

Elimination and pelvic signals: Urge to urinate or defecate, bladder fullness, pelvic pressure or discomfort, menstrual cramping or heaviness, ovulation-related sensations

Immune and inflammatory signals: General feelings of being unwell or "off," achiness, malaise, feverish sensations, illness-related fatigue, tenderness in lymph nodes

Skin and surface sensations: Touch, pressure, tingling, prickling, itching, crawling sensations, warmth or coolness on the skin

Energy and arousal levels: Sleepiness, fatigue, sluggishness, alertness, jitteriness, hyperarousal, startle responses, sense of internal speed (slow or fast)

Emotional body cues: Chest tightness or heaviness, "butterflies" in the stomach, warmth or expansion in the chest, sinking or dropping sensations, internal pressure, agitation, trembling, tension patterns linked with emotions

Research has also found a moderate to strong link between dissociation and *alexithymia*, which involves difficulty recognizing and articulating feelings or needs (Reyno et al., 2020), as well as difficulty with consciously feeling and articulating the emotional experience of chronic pain. Parts with unarticulated emotional pain may use the body to get attention and support by bringing attention to their physical symptoms, talking about them, or even exacerbating them or triggering them. We can help clients with these parts by focusing on whatever they present and getting to know them with Self-energy. Since people who are alexithymic don't recognize feelings and don't connect the physical experience of emotion with words, they can more easily identify feelings and needs by looking at a written list when offered the possibility. In appendix B, we've included an open access list of words from the Center for Nonviolent Communication that can help clients describe feelings and needs.

Nonetheless, dissociation, like many skills, can also be beneficial. The IFS process, for example, involves purposeful dissociation. We move from one time zone (the external present) to another (an internal two-way, time-travel freeway) via a natural dissociative trance state that most people find easy to access. In IFS, we call this *going inside*. We leave the external present and its material constraints to travel within an internal plane of existence. Here, time travel is the norm and past experiences are only concluded when the parts who are stuck there can leave.

Charting a New Path Forward

As we saw with Tina's dissociative TV watching and comfort-eating, as well as Ronan's aggression, chronic stress disrupts people's internal systems into adulthood. In this state, the autonomic nervous, heart, neuroendocrine, and immune systems cannot return to optimal functioning. Nonemergency processes like digestion, growth, and reproduction are put on hold. All this activation speaks of protective parts who are in continual crisis because they no longer trust their capacity to deal with challenges. Eventually, extreme inhibition leads to rebellion. For example, Tina lived in lonely despair, comforting herself until she was ill, while Ronan lived in lonely terror, oscillating between fleeing, fighting, and freezing.

When reactive firefighters break social norms, managers get upset and become critical. The clash between Ronan's critical manager and his rageful firefighter is a good example. Inner conflict activates the limbic system—a.k.a. the "emotional brain"—increasing its sensitivity to threats via neuroception. As critical managers shame firefighter parts, exiles become reactive and make their way to consciousness. We see this in Ronan's stomachaches, headaches, and sleep disturbance, all of which started in childhood when he was being bullied after school. Whenever he felt stressed, Ronan had difficulty thinking, and his reactions to feeling shameful became more intense. He described it this way: "When things are hard and I feel like a failure, I'm at my worst. My brain doesn't work. I hate myself. I go through weeks of terrible headaches and stomachaches every day and can't sleep because I'm obsessing about the stupid things I did or said. No one understands. It's just horrible."

The Brain on Stress

Prolonged or overwhelming challenges harm the brain. Three brain regions are especially vulnerable:

1. The limbic system, particularly the amygdala, which regulates emotions and processes fear and danger
2. The hippocampus, where learning circuits develop early on
3. The prefrontal cortex, which governs impulse control, attention, complex thought, organization, and problem-solving

When stress compromises higher thought processes, our primitive brain circuits take over (van der Kolk, 2014; Woo et al., 2021). This can lead to repetitive negative thinking and worry, catastrophizing, rumination, self-blame, and the blaming of others (Flores-Kanter et al., 2021). From an IFS perspective, these are the behaviors of fearful, stressed protectors. The key to minimizing the negative impacts of stress on our physical and emotional health is to recover and return to an emotionally regulated state. We introduce a new, more accepting and appreciative perspective on the activities of parts coping with burdened systems. In particular, we point out the protective nature of negative emotions, thoughts, and beliefs, and offer them hope for a new path forward. ▌

[CHAPTER 5]

IFS Health Therapy Phase 1: Step-by-Step with Protectors

IFS health treatment can be divided into three phases. In the initial phase of IFS treatment, our primary task is to help the protective system feel less afraid and more willing to allow access to exiles. As therapy progresses and change is integrated into the client's life, our focus on relational support expands beyond the office.

- **Phase 1: Building trust and encouraging protectors to unblend.** First, we befriend the client's protective system, find out which ones are involved with the client's physical illness, offer them a healing path, and address their fears. We aim to show protectors how treatment can proceed safely and, ultimately, access vulnerable exiles.
- **Phase 2: Unburdening and healing exiles in steps.** Next, exiles show or tell their stories, regulate physiologically in relationship with the Self, and release their burdens.
- **Phase 3: Integration and creating a more balanced life.** Here, we focus on liberating protectors from unmanageable responsibilities and extreme roles. As protectors integrate the good news that Self is here to take responsibility and hurt parts are not defective, they shift from fear-driven roles to developmentally appropriate interests and pursuits. The Self is now available to take the lead on how to spend time (e.g., creatively, spiritually, or in work and play), who to spend time with, how to handle money, how to stay present, and what the body needs for food, sleep, exercise, and relaxation. This phase shifts the developmental journey from chronic stress and illness to a life of enriching pursuits and nourishing relationships, inside and out.

You have witnessed some early stages of this process in the dialogues described so far. Protectors like Tina's and Ronan's were tasked with keeping the stressed system balanced and functioning internally despite illness, burdens, disagreements, and the ever-present troubles of the outside. Protective parts need to feel hope and trust in our plan for healing. They want to know that the Self of the client (and the therapist!) won't make things worse and can deliver on this idea of freedom from stress. Like all of us, protective parts develop trust through experience. When they encounter the Self-energy of the client and clinician, hear the hopeful but realistic plan for their freedom, and see that their fears can be addressed, they cooperate. We ask them to unblend and allow contact between the client's Self and their exiles. Negotiations with protectors can be straightforward if things go smoothly.

Therefore, we start with protectors, getting to know them in a trust-building process—with both us and the client's Self—to address their concerns and fears. We begin with any symptom or part on the chronic stress cycle and, as you saw in the dialogue with Tina in the previous chapter, proceed with the 6 F's:

1. **Find:** Ask how the client notices the symptom or part (e.g., physical sensations, images, emotions, thoughts, beliefs, or behavior).

2. **Focus on it:** If it's a symptom, focus on it like you would a part. Ask the client to focus on it and notice more about it (e.g., physical sensations, emotions, or thoughts that accompany the symptoms).

3. **Feel toward:** Check for qualities of Self-energy (as evidenced by the 8 C's) by asking, "How do you feel toward [*the part*]?"

   a. If it's a protector (e.g., judgmental, anxious, skeptical), acknowledge its effort and ask if it is willing to relax. (If not, it becomes the new target part.)

   b. Once it softens, check again for qualities of the Self: "How do you feel toward the part now?"

4. **Befriend:** Once the client feels curious, calm, appreciative, and so on, establish a relationship between the Self and the part.

   - "Is the part aware of your [*e.g., curiosity, calm, appreciation*]?"
   - "Invite it to take in that [*e.g., curiosity, compassion, appreciation*]."
   - "If it didn't have this job, what would it rather do instead?"

5. **Flesh out:** Once there's a relational connection, find out more about the part's role:

   - What is its job?
   - What is it hoping to accomplish?
   - When did it take on this role?
   - What is it afraid would happen if it didn't fulfill this role?

6. **Address its fears:** If the target part fears that another protector or an exile will blend, address its fears and gain permission to connect with the exiled part by asking:

   - "Would it help you if we could help this protector be less extreme?"
   - "Would it get you off the hook if we could heal this vulnerable part safely?"
   - "Would it help if we could find out what needs to change so that this part no longer has to keep [*e.g., giving you headaches, working this hard, being so scared or tense*]?"

Working with Protectors Step-by-Step

To illustrate how these steps look in practice, you'll meet another client, Leonie, who had a history of childhood trauma, struggled with anxiety and depression, and had a serious autoimmune disease. We often find this combination in relation to chronic illness. Leonie, an Irish American woman in her late 20s, was the younger of two siblings. She came to IFS health therapy seeking help for unremitting anxiety. In the initial meeting, she mentioned having had Crohn's disease since she was a teenager. This affects the digestive tract, causing inflammation, intestinal infections, abscesses and ulcers, and chronic pain. Leonie had experienced long periods of remission, but about six months before her first therapy appointment, the Crohn's flared. Her physical symptoms included abdominal cramps and pain, fatigue, diarrhea, blood in her stools, and weight loss. She had also developed some of the less common symptoms of Crohn's disease, including tenderness and redness in her eyes and a rash on her shins. Her biologic medication had stopped working, and a new medication wasn't helping either. Fearing that she would need to be hospitalized again, she gave her therapist and doctor consent to communicate.

Leonie: My anxiety has been worse than ever. I think it's affecting my Crohn's symptoms. Is that possible?

Therapist: Sure. Psychological stress, which we can think of as parts dealing with stress inside and out, can exacerbate Crohn's symptoms and contribute to flares.

Leonie: What does that mean for me?

Therapist: Let's ask parts who feel anxious and stressed what they've been doing to cope.

Leonie: But what's the connection between my parts and Crohn's disease? And how can therapy help?

> Realizing that a part of Leonie wants to hear the therapist's perspective, the therapist uses implicit direct access (speaking to a part directly without naming it as a part) to do some psychoeducation.

Therapist: When your parts stress, the immune system in your gut activates, which can lead to inflammation and Crohn's symptoms. The negative beliefs and feelings that these parts hold affect your body and mood, and their coping strategies affect, for example, your sleep and eating. In therapy, we help the parts and their stress levels go down.

Leonie: Like, I could go back into remission?

Therapist: If we help stressed, anxious parts feel better, your body will feel better. We'll see if that leads to remission.

> Offering realistic hope, not promises

Leonie: Okay. Is there something I can do between sessions?

Therapist: Do you want things to do between sessions?

Leonie: Kind of . . . maybe.

Therapist: Sounds like some of your parts have different preferences.

Leonie: Oh. [*Pauses to think it over.*] That's probably true.

Therapist: Do you have a journal?

Leonie: I use one sometimes.

Therapist: When and if you feel up for it, you could start noticing this anxious part and what it's thinking and feeling, along with other parts, like those who don't want to journal. But no pressure!

> Building trust by recognizing and offering flexibility to different parts

Leonie: If I do journal, should I bring it to our sessions?

Therapist: Only if you want to.

Leonie: Okay.

> Sensing that some parts were looking for reliable support, while other parts didn't want to feel bossed around, Leonie's therapist continued to model flexibility and offer choices based on preference in place of "shoulds."

Therapist: If you want to share anything, I'm totally interested. But I'm hearing parts with different opinions. [*Leonie nods.*] Can they let journaling be completely free of obligations and "shoulds"? If it feels good and right, try it. See how it goes.

Leonie: I like the idea of deciding based on what feels good and right and whether I like it rather than feeling I *should* do it.

Therapist: That would be a new approach to decisions.

Leonie: Totally. I never think about what feels good and right for me. [*The therapist makes a note.*] Is that another part?

Therapist: [*Encouraging Leonie to be a parts detector*] What do you think? [*Leonie nods.*] Good catch.

Leonie: But they all just feel like me.

Therapist: That's because they *are* parts of you.

Leonie started tracking her parts in a journal. In the next session, she brought her journal and shared what she had been noticing. The following dialogue illustrates a variety of potential sticking points and distractions. The therapist's interventions nudge Leonie back on track.

Leonie: I'm noticing that anxious part and its worries in my journal. It helps to think of it as just one part of me.

Therapist: Good. Is our plan to learn more about stressors that affect the anxious part, and to get to know more about it, still right for today?

> Recalling where the last session left off, the therapist checks with the client about priorities.

LEONIE: [*Breaks eye contact and looks down.*]

Sensing another part and knowing that Leonie needs a calm, attuned presence, the therapist pauses and then notices the tension in her own shoulders. Internally, the therapist tells her tense part, "I feel you in my shoulders. Can you let me handle this?" She takes a breath. Her shoulders relax and she responds to this new part of Leonie, using direct access to check in.

THERAPIST: Are you okay? [*A pause, waiting for Leonie to respond.*]

LEONIE: I felt hopeful after the last session, but my Crohn's symptoms are still high and so is my anxiety. I feel awful.

The therapist notices that Leonie's language keeps changing. Sometimes she refers to the anxious part as "it" and sometimes she uses "I," which indicates that she is moving in and out of the part. The therapist follows her lead using the words *you, it,* or *this anxious part.*

THERAPIST: How are you feeling right now?

Using implicit direct access

LEONIE: I'm scared. I'm still scared so much of the time not knowing what's going to happen next.

THERAPIST: I can understand that, given the symptoms you experience. Is there more you want to say about the anxiety of this part right now?

Transitioning back to insight

LEONIE: If we get to know more about this part and its fear, can we help it with the anxiety?

THERAPIST: Yes. Let's learn more about what it fears. That will tell us where to go next. Is that a good plan for today?

LEONIE: Yeah.

Having determined their plan was still relevant, Leonie and her therapist have contracted to continue learning what the anxious part fears. The following dialogue illustrates how Leonie and her therapist followed through with this plan, representing the first phase of IFS health therapy.

Start with the target part (a protector or symptom) identified on the chronic stress cycle.

THERAPIST: Let's get to know the part of you who feels anxious much of the time.

LEONIE: Okay.

Find: Ask how the client notices the part.

THERAPIST: How are you aware of this part? For example, you might notice it in your body or your thoughts.

LEONIE: I've been shaking with anxiety all day.

Focus: Have the client focus on the part.

THERAPIST: As you focus on that shakiness, what thoughts, feelings, sensations, or images come up?

LEONIE: It's like, "I can't stand this disease. I want it to stop. This is scary. I never know what's going to happen next!"

Feel toward: Ask how they feel toward the part to check for qualities of Self.

THERAPIST: And as you notice that shakiness and those thoughts, how do you feel toward the part?

LEONIE: I totally understand why it's anxious! I get it!

Befriend: Once the client feels curious, calm, compassionate, or another quality of the Self, help them get to connect with the part.

THERAPIST: Let it know that you understand. [*Leonie looks puzzled, so the therapist attunes to the need and offers more specific options.*] You can use words, use touch, or communicate telepathically or through the senses—whatever works best for this part.

LEONIE: Okay. [*Focusing inside*] She could feel that!

THERAPIST: What did you do?

LEONIE: She's a young teen—in middle school—so I reached out and put my hand on her shoulder.

THERAPIST: How did she respond?

LEONIE: She was surprised, but she could sense my understanding.

Flesh out: Help the client find out more about the part and its fears.

THERAPIST: That's great, Leonie. What is she hoping to accomplish with all the worry?

LEONIE: She's trying to stop something bad from happening, like someone getting mad.

THERAPIST: What would happen if someone got mad?

Another part of Leonie: Could I be making this all up?

THERAPIST: Is that another part?

LEONIE: Yeah. That thought just popped up.

THERAPIST: What do you say to it?

LEONIE: It's okay. It moved over there [*motioning to the side*] to watch.

THERAPIST: Okay. Go back to the middle school girl. What is she afraid would happen if someone got mad?

LEONIE: [*After a pause*] She's worried that something bad will happen. People will yell and be terrible.

THERAPIST: Do you know what she's talking about, Leonie?

The therapist trusts the client's Self to understand.

Leonie: Yeah, I do.

Therapist: Let her know.

Coming back to the Self-to-part relationship and reinforcing their connection

Leonie: Yeah. She's glad I understand.

Therapist: Does she protect another part?

Leonie: [*After a long pause*] She does. There's a part that's afraid of anger and people fighting.

Therapist: How is it for you to hear this, Leonie?

Checking for triggered parts

Leonie: I'm okay. It's not totally shocking. This is my family.

Address its fears: If the target part fears that another protector or an exile will blend, address its fear.

Therapist: If we could help the scared, anxious part, would she still feel frightened and need to be vigilant?

Leonie: If we could do that without anything bad happening, she'd be relieved. But she doubts it's possible and she's afraid of making things worse.

Therapist: Does that make sense to you?

Leonie: It does!

Therapist: What does she want you to know about making things worse?

Leonie: She's afraid of a big rift with my parents. She worries about all the anger. I've always been the peacekeeper in my family. My father and my older brother have bad tempers. I hold people together. Maybe that's why I'm sick.

Therapist: Does the peacekeeper part believe it's *you* who's angry?

Leonie: [*Chuckles.*] The peacekeeper is a part? How would I know if she thinks it's me who's angry?

Therapist: Is she afraid?

Leonie: Yes. This is the worried girl. Anger is bad.

Therapist: Is she worried about an angry part of you?

Leonie: It seems like she's worried about *me* getting angry and making things worse.

Therapist: What would happen if you got angry?

Leonie: Girls don't get angry. Not in my family. Women don't lose control. They'd shame me and I'd be alone.

Therapist: Did that happen?

Leonie: Of course.

THERAPIST: Is she protecting the part who got shamed and feels alone?

LEONIE: Yes.

THERAPIST: Do you know that part, Leonie?

LEONIE: Sort of. Not strongly. But I believe it.

THERAPIST: Will the worried girl let us help that part?

LEONIE: Only if it doesn't take over.

THERAPIST: We'll ask it not to overwhelm. It doesn't have to take over to be heard.

LEONIE: Okay.

Here is Leonie's working parts map, created during the session just described.

Leonie's Initial Parts Map

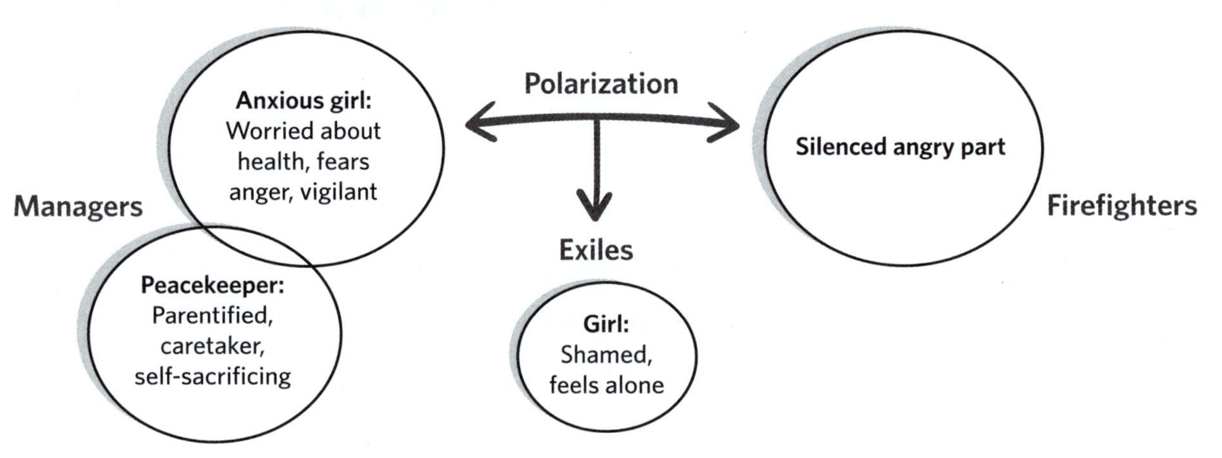

Silently Communicating with Our Own Parts as Therapists

When Leonie's IFS health therapist first heard her story, including the gut-wrenching pain of Crohn's disease that involved sores, fissures, and inflammation, some parts of the therapist became anxious. Her neck and shoulders tensed, and she was filled with a sense of urgency. When a part takes over in us during a session, we need quick internal action, and we can communicate with our parts silently inside despite being with other people. Sometimes, a part needs reassurance (*This is a lot to take in! I feel your fear!*). Sometimes, the part needs telepathic understanding (*I know! I see that too!*). And sometimes, it needs a physical response, like placing your hand on a tense muscle or adjusting your posture. Here is how Leonie's therapist helped her parts unblend with an internal exchange followed by a physical action.

1. **Ask a part for breathing room:** You may want to ask your parts for breathing room during a session. Leonie's therapist noticed tension in her shoulders and neck as she was listening. Inside, she

said, *I feel your tension and concern. If you open up some room for me, I can take some breaths with you. This isn't your job. I'll talk with Leonie about her illness.*

2. **Breathe with your parts:** You then consciously co-regulate with your parts by taking a few deep breaths with them. This allows your parts to release tension, and their need for internal conversation will typically recede quickly. When your parts know and trust you, it only takes a few shared breaths to help them unblend, which makes more room for your Self-energy. Co-regulating breathing is also a handy skill to share with clients.

Experiential Exercise: Breathing Room

This is a practice for helping your parts relax and feel safe with the Self. We recommend first practicing this in a quiet, safe place before attempting it in more stressful circumstances. You will notice a natural shift in the mind-body as parts and the nervous system relax.

Step 1: Orient the target part for a comfortable mind-body experience with your Self.

- Invite the activated part to look around and take in the environment for safety.
- Make any helpful adjustments (lighting, temperature, support for the body, sound level, privacy, or anything else needed for your parts and body to relax).
- Sit or lie somewhere comfortable with your spine supported.

Step 2: Tune in to the part by shifting your attention inward.

- Allow the external world to drift into the background as you focus inside.
- See how the activated part is showing up in your mind-body.
- Notice what's happening in your thoughts, emotions, and physical sensations: fear, tension, shaking, pain, anger, anxiety, tightness, fogginess, restlessness, or anything else.

Step 3: Breathe with the part.

- Ask the part to open some breathing room for you inside.
- Take an inhale together, followed by a comfortable, slow exhale.
- Continue for as long as feels right for you and your part, without trying to change anything.
- Let your mind-body notice and register, "I am safe here."

As you and your part breathe together, mental and physiological shifts will naturally occur as you settle into co-regulation. In your Self, you are the calm, non-anxious presence who is needed by your parts.

As a therapist, how do you notice your parts? For example, do you notice them as feelings (e.g., dislike, distress, alarm), physical sensations (e.g., sleepiness, a stomachache, discomfort in your chair), or thoughts (e.g., *I wish this session would end* or *I wonder what I'm having for dinner*)? Take a moment to think about how your parts manifest in your mind-body. Here's an easy rule: If it's not the Self, it's a part. Therefore, before you worry about recognizing how parts can manifest in session, focus on the distinct experience of embodying Self and being Self-led. When you are in Self, you will experience the 8 C's: compassion, courage, clarity, curiosity, connectedness, creativity, calm, and confidence. To these, we would also add some non-C qualities, like kindness and love. Similarly, in this state, you will embody Self-leadership with the 5 P's: presence, playfulness, perspective, patience, and persistence.

In addition to tuning in for these qualities of the Self, here are some questions that can help you identify your parts (Sowell, 2020). If you answer *no* to these questions, it's a part.

Discerning the Presence of a Part

Notice your thoughts and feelings:	Notice your body:
• Is your mind open? • Are your thoughts clear? • Are you curious? • Do you feel connected to your immediate environment? To other people? • Do you feel accepting of yourself and others? • Is your heart open? • Are you communicating calm, curiosity, interest, or understanding?	• Does it feel safe to be in your body? • Is your body calm? • Can you sit quietly without needing to move? • Is it okay to be seen by other people? • Are your shoulders, jaw, neck, and stomach relaxed? • Are you breathing with ease? Inhaling and exhaling at a comfortable pace? • Is your voice calm and modulated?

By recognizing and attending to your own parts, you are able to extend Self-energy to your clients as well. This can be especially powerful for clients who were not offered consistent Self-energy or co-regulation from their caregivers in childhood, leading to the development of legacy burdens. We will explore one such burden, parentification, as we continue Leonie's story in the following section.

The Legacy Burden of Parentification

In the previous vignette, the therapist asked Leonie what would happen if she got angry, and a part answered by saying that girls don't get angry or lose control in her family, as they are otherwise shamed and shunned. This statement revealed several protector fears and beliefs that were perpetuating Leonie's chronic stress:

- Anger is bad, hurts people, and causes problems.
- When someone gets mad, something bad will happen.
- If I were to get mad at my parents, they would punish and shame me.

- An angry part of me could come out, take over, and make things worse.
- My system could be overwhelmed by the exile's emotional pain.
- I can't be angry; I have to keep the peace and hold the family together.

Recall from chapter 2 that in IFS, these are called inherited (or *legacy*) burdens, which can be cultural and familial. Some of Leonie's parts were loyal to this family belief that angry girls are bad and shameful. Because her nominal adult caretakers had hurt her and her brother during childhood, Leonie's managers became *parentified* early on. They fawned, appeased, and made sure Leonie acted like a responsible grown-up, which included not feeling angry and not asking anyone to attend to her needs. Her protective parts adopted the gender-based legacy bias that angry girls are shameful, bad, and unlovable, and when an angry young firefighter rebelled, Leonie was indeed criticized and rejected by her family.

For example, when Leonie entered treatment with a flare of Crohn's disease, she was struggling to maintain her full-time job, yet she and her mother both expected her to be available for caretaking on a daily basis. Every day, Leonie dutifully checked in with her mother and her brother, Nick, who had pulled away from the family after years of tension with their father. Rather than feeling exploited by this situation, Leonie wanted to support her brother and felt pity for her mother, who she described as trapped and submissive toward her critical, explosive father. When Leonie's father would depart abruptly after a rageful outburst, he, too, expected Leonie to come to her mother's rescue. When he returned hours or days later, none of them would speak of the incident or his behavior. Leonie's peacekeeper also feared that internal healing would unleash a firefighter who wanted to abandon the project of rescuing her parents. By protecting the status quo to prevent this dreaded outcome, it prolonged her exiles' banishment and further damaged her body. Often, parentified parts can't resolve the dilemma of loyalty without help.

Leonie and her therapist needed to appreciate the inherited gifts of her family's cultural roots, including their celebration of an individual's contribution to the common good of family and community. On the other hand, Leonie needed to recognize and let go of the inherited burden of extreme self-reliance, which had harmed her, her family, and her community. Accordingly, she needed to sort the burdens of her parentified role from the values-based behaviors she wished to continue. In the following example, Leonie's therapist asks questions about culture and values to help her with this sorting. This dialogue occurred after Leonie's brief check-in at the beginning of the session. She was feeling physically worse after going to her parents' house the night before and staying with her mother at the end of a draining workday. She had received a text from her father telling her to go to their house and be with her mother. Leonie disclosed that she thought he had probably raged and walked out, leaving her mother alone and upset.

LEONIE: Before I got my father's text, I wanted to go straight home after work. But I couldn't say no.

THERAPIST: Were there cultural or family messages that made it hard for you to stick with your plan?

LEONIE: My commitment to the common good is confusing at times like this, when my Crohn's is flaring and I need to take care of myself.

THERAPIST: *Contributing* to the common good is a beautiful legacy, but living it as an absolute *commitment* could be burdensome.

Leonie: It is! And the belief that self-sacrifice is honorable and taking care of yourself is selfish, at least for the women in the family, doesn't help. There's also pride in self-reliance and the message "family takes care of family," which means it's okay to count on family but nobody else. Wow, there's a lot of these messages! "What goes on in this house stays in this house!"

Therapist: Are there values that you hold that conflict with those beliefs and expectations?

Leonie: I'm not great at accepting help, but I think it's how we're meant to be living. I think I could get well again if I could take better care of my health—not just by eating and exercising well, but by resting when my body hurts. I need to connect more with my Self, my friends and community, and my extended family.

Therapist: Are you noticing parts coming up as we're talking about this, Leonie?

Leonie: I notice the tension between what I've been saying and the messages about duty and taking care of my mother so that she'll feel like I'm a good daughter and not be upset with me.

Therapist: Check inside to see who's talking.

Leonie: It's the part who keeps the peace. She feels good when my mother approves of her.

Therapist: How are you feeling toward her as you listen inside?

Leonie: I understand how she feels and how important it is to her to be there for my mother and for Nick.

Therapist: Is she noticing how well you are understanding her feelings and needs?

Therapist: She appreciates my understanding, but she's focused on my mother.

Therapist: Is there more you're noticing?

Leonie: The anxious part is worrying about the Crohn's getting worse if things don't change.

Therapist: How are you feeling toward that worried part as we're talking?

Leonie: I understand. I know how hard and scary this disease is.

Therapist: Is it aware of your compassion and understanding?

Leonie: She likes that I'm here and talking about this. She wants to feel more secure.

Therapist: Of course she does. When we're processing legacy burdens, it feels good to remember what has sustained us too. Are there traditions or family legacies that could help you feel more connected to your culture, your Self, and your parts?

Leonie: Humor comes to mind! The banter that I grew up with in my extended family was great. But the love of music in my family is what I treasure the most. I used to listen to music all the time. I love everything—the hymns and traditional Irish music, the ballads and pop music that I grew up with. It's good to remember that I still have it!

Therapist: For sure. Music is an incredible inheritance!

Leonie: The best!

In our experience, clients with chronic illnesses are more likely to locate parts who have *traumatic bonds*, meaning they are emotionally attached to unsafe or unavailable caregivers who enlist the child to take care of them. Neglected parts long for attention and love (Dariotis et al., 2023). Parentified parts respond to this unrequited longing by appeasing and accommodating powerful people (Sweezy, 2023). Leonie, for example, learned to ignore feeling angry about her parents' boundary violations, which had the unintended consequence of diminishing her sense of agency in social settings. She also became unaware of her body, her parts, and her Self because her needs threatened her parents and their status quo. This set her up for a cascade of negative health consequences.

Since parentified parts are loyal caretakers of dysfunctional parents and may view their sacrifices as evidence of strength and resilience, we recommend exploring their consequences with curiosity and understanding. These parts fear differentiating from the family and being alone in the world. Leonie's parts, for example, were terrified of disclosing the reality of life in her family. Whenever a client's Self begins to recognize parental transgressions such as these and the cost of their protective efforts to the mind-body, their parentified parts will need a lot of support and appreciation.

Affect Phobia Breeds Polarization

Leonie's parentification and avoidance of anger is a good example of how a negative bias about any emotion prolongs internal stress and causes protectors to polarize. This avoidance of specific emotions is called an *affect phobia*, a term that speaks to how protective parts panic in response to banned feelings (McCullough et al., 2003). Affect phobias illustrate polarizations between the following parts: (1) those who inhibit spontaneity and risk to prevent negative feelings, and (2) those who disinhibit by engaging in various costly behaviors to soothe or distract from negative feelings. Indeed, Leonie and her therapist identified several of these polarized protectors who were maintaining her costly status quo. These protectors were evident by the following verbal and cognitive signs of affect phobia and polarization:

1. **Negative beliefs about anger:**
   - "Girls don't get angry. Anger is bad."
   - "When someone gets mad, something bad will happen."
   - "Getting mad will only makes things worse."
2. **Traumatic bonds:**
   - "When my mother needs my support, I feel like I'm important."
   - "When my father counts on me to take care of my mother, I feel like I matter."
   - "Helping my parents and being needed feels better than counting on them to take care of me."
3. **Self-shaming and self-sacrifice indicated by "shoulds" and "should-nots":**
   - "I shouldn't talk back. I should be loyal and watch what I say outside the family."
   - "I shouldn't be selfish. I should help my parents and do my part."

Unfortunately, Leonie's body was paying the price for being too nice to set limits, which is a notable observation of patients with chronic autoimmune diseases (Hughes & Hunter, 2022; Russell et al., 2016). That is, these patients tend to inhibit anger, as we anecdotally observed during the IFS rheumatoid arthritis study (Shadick et al., 2013). This shame-based inhibition of negative feelings has been linked to chronic physical as well as mental illness (Chapman et al., 2013; Maté, 2022; Moriarity & Slavich, 2023). Indeed, Leonie noticed that the stress with her family preceded the flare-up of her Crohn's disease. A protector who was angry about this and concerned about her health had recently disclosed that her father, an upstanding citizen and nice guy in their community, was shaming, controlling, and rageful at home. Her peacekeeper part, like her mother's, who was a loyal caretaker for her parents, appeased him. In the following dialogue, Leonie is feeling guilty about disclosing this family secret to her therapist.

Throughout this dialogue, the therapist introduces IFS health therapy concepts like affect phobia and polarization, answers questions about illness and causal factors, links somatic manifestations of emotion to Leonie's unfolding story, and ends the session with the next session in mind. The therapist wants Leonie to notice parts who are polarized between anger and guilt. You will see the therapist take the following steps to do so: (1) identify the somatic manifestations of the conflict between parts, and (2) understand both sides.

Leonie: I've been having a lot of belly cramps. I feel guilty that I told you about my father's anger.

> Her Crohn's symptoms have been flaring.

Therapist: I'm sorry to hear about the cramping. Has talking honestly with me about your father been on your mind since the last session?

Leonie: Yeah. I don't usually talk about it. My mother acts like everything's fine around people.

Therapist: So, telling me about your father's rage was new? [*Leonie nods.*] And a part feels guilty about that?

Leonie: It's the peacekeeper. I never want to trigger my father.

> Leonie names the peacekeeper part, indicating some separation, but then speaks from the part, using the pronoun "I."

Therapist: What's that like for you?

> The therapist continues using implicit direct access with the guilty peacekeeper part.

Leonie: I feel guilty, like I betrayed my mother. I always feel sorry for her and try to make her life easier. [*She crosses her arms over her belly and curls forward slightly.*]

> Leonie's peacekeeping part believes the part who disclosed her father's behavior was betraying her long-silent mother.

Therapist: Do you notice what's happening physically as you speak about this, Leonie?

> The therapist notices Leonie is starting to curl up around her belly and asks an open-ended question aimed at bringing Leonie's attention to her body.

Leonie: [*Closes her eyes and focuses inward.*] My belly is churning. I'm afraid my mother will be mad at me. I have a part who *wanted* to tell you about my dad. [*Opens her eyes and looks up at the therapist.*]

Leonie's peacekeeping part speaks as if her mother knows she has divulged forbidden information.

Therapist: This is hard. [*Leonie nods.*] Let me know if I've got it right. One part of you [*holding up one hand*] tries to keep the peace and fears your mother's anger. It feels guilty because another part spoke openly about your father's rage. [*Leonie nods.*] On the other hand [*holding up the other hand*], there is another part of you who *wanted* to expose your father's behavior. The peacekeeper feels obliged to maintain secrets, but this other part doesn't want to do that anymore.

Offering Leonie a visual representing the polarized parts while describing their different strategies

Leonie: That's it. My mother is trapped. She makes excuses for my father all the time. "Your father works so hard. He's stressed."

Therapist: Does that make you angry?

Hearing anger, the therapist names the feeling of the part.

Leonie: [*A long pause.*] Maybe. [*Another long pause before Leonie blurts out*] My father is a bully, and my mother pretends everything is fine!

Therapist: This is the part who wants to tell the truth now. [*Leonie nods.*] What is that like for the peacekeeper?

Tracking Leonie's parts as they arise

Leonie: Painful. Scary.

Therapist: Leonie, your mother isn't here with us, right?

Leonie: Right.

Therapist: Does the peacekeeper know that?

Leonie: Not really.

Therapist: Let her know our conversations are private. Your parts can say anything here and then work on a consensus about what to say outside of here.

Updating a part who is stuck in the past

Leonie: [*Sounding relieved*] That's good. She likes that.

Therapist: We can hear and understand both of these disagreeing parts.

Leonie: Does this have something to do with the stomach cramps?

Therapist: Research shows that stress does affect the gut, but we won't know if or how much it's affecting you right now without asking.

LEONIE: Asking who?

THERAPIST: The peacekeeper has been in a conflict with other parts for a long time, maybe especially with this angry part. Is that right?

LEONIE: [*Nodding*] The "keep the peace" part is me.

THERAPIST: It *is* you much of the time. The peacekeeper has taken responsibility for you and all your other parts. Do you see how that makes sense, given your history?

LEONIE: In my family, only my father gets to be angry. When my brother pushed back, they told him to leave.

THERAPIST: You've described your father's rage ruling the roost. When you got angry, he shamed you. And when your brother got angry, he was kicked out. Of course, kids are afraid when adults misuse anger! But we need our anger. Angry parts tell us when people are stepping on our toes. When we feel comfortable being proactive about setting limits with other people, angry protectors don't have to work so hard.

LEONIE: But I don't feel angry, so I can't set limits.

The peacekeeper chimes in.

THERAPIST: Would the peacekeeper, who doesn't get angry, be willing to sit down right now with you and the angry part?

LEONIE: She doesn't want to.

THERAPIST: Because?

LEONIE: She's scared the angry part will take over.

THERAPIST: Does she see you?

LEONIE: Yes.

THERAPIST: Who does the peacekeeper think you are?

LEONIE: A little kid.

THERAPIST: Ask the little kid to sit right next to you and have her look again. [*Pauses.*] Who does she see now?

An unblending request

LEONIE: She's surprised. She sees me.

THERAPIST: What do you say to her?

LEONIE: I'm here to help both of you.

THERAPIST: Is she willing?

LEONIE: Yes, tentatively.

Therapist: Tentative is fine. Invite her to speak up if she's concerned about something. Okay? [*Leonie nods.*] Great. Who needs your attention first?

The Self in Leonie and the therapist help polarized parts navigate their relationship

Leonie: The angry part wants to speak. He says, "You never listen! You're stupid—"

Therapist: Oops! No insults. Okay? We want him to be heard. What is it like for him when no one listens?

Leonie's Angry Part: Terrible! I warn her. I tell her the truth, but she doesn't listen.

The angry part chimes in directly, expressing his frustration.

Therapist: She's listening now. What's that like for you?

The therapist responds to the angry part directly, not asking Leonie to be the intermediary.

Leonie's Angry Part: [*Grudgingly*] Better.

Therapist: If Leonie could keep both of you safe, would you need to be so angry?

Leonie's Angry Part: No.

Negotiating a truce

Therapist: Okay. Leonie, let's talk with the peacekeeper. Did she hear what the angry part said?

Returning to insight, in which the therapist talks with the client's Self, who is in direct communication with parts

Leonie: She did. She feels bad. She says she was just trying to help.

Therapist: What do you say to her?

Leonie: I know that's true. I appreciate her. She's worked so hard!

Offering appreciation

Therapist: And back when you had no choices, peacekeeping was a good option for being safe, wasn't it?

Leonie: It was.

Suggesting a way of understanding past circumstances and the extreme roles of protectors

Therapist: But now . . .

Leonie: Now things are different.

Therapist: Does she hear you? [*Leonie nods.*] Is she willing to get to know you better to find out if you can help?

Leonie: Yes.

Contrasting the past with present circumstances

Therapist: Who does she protect?

Leonie: Everyone!

Therapist: What does she need from you right now?

Leonie: She needs thanks. She needs to know she's not bad.

Identifying a part's need

Therapist: She is very good! She worked hard. She helped. She is clever and smart. Can the angry part see her perspective?

Affirming a part's worth and good intentions

Leonie: Yeah. But he wants an apology.

Therapist: From her or you?

Leonie: Me.

Therapist: What do you say to him?

Leonie: I'm so sorry! It wasn't your fault. I wish I had been there to help. You were totally right to be angry, but the peacekeeper was also right that it was dangerous to get mad back then.

Therapist: [*A pause.*] How does he respond?

Leonie: He says, "Okay."

Leonie's Self acknowledging and offering to help both parts in the polarization

Therapist: Good. What else does he need?

Leonie: He's okay for now.

Therapist: So, let me sum up. See if this sounds accurate. Your father's rage ruled the roost. [*Leonie nods.*] But when you got angry, you were shamed, and when your brother got angry, he was expelled. [*She nods again.*] So, the peacekeeper kept you safe by silencing the angry part, and the angry part has been feeling frustrated and dissed. But now they understand each other and see that you're here to help.

Leonie: Yes.

Therapist: How did all this affect your body?

Leonie: I know you say it affected my body, but I never put that together.

Therapist: When I'm angry, scared, or sad, like you, I feel it. Feelings are information. When challenging things happen, our parts give us a lot of information through feelings, which start in the body. And if these parts eventually take action, their behavior also affects the body.

Leonie: Okay. I think these stomach cramps are more about feeling afraid than angry.

Therapist: Afraid of?

Leonie: [*Pauses, then chuckles.*] Anger. Okay, I get it!

Therapist: Sounds like that conflict between the peacekeeper and the angry part plays out in your gut. Some other things, like diet and medication, could also be affecting your gut.

Leonie: Well, the conflict has stopped.

Therapist: Great. Are they willing to be more direct with you? They don't need to keep fighting to get your attention and adding to your stress.

Leonie: They're saying maybe. If I get the cramps again, I'll know to check in with them.

Therapist: When their conflict stirs up your cramps, you'll know they need your help. But eventually they'll find that being direct and asking for help is less work than causing you pain.

By now, Leonie was openhearted with her parts and curious about their experiences. In this session, she saw how the two sides of a long-standing conflict between guilt and anger were linked to her physical symptoms. Of course, the session also pinpointed the big problem of the current stress of her relationships with her parents. Aware that this problem would require Self-leadership from Leonie to prevent her protectors from getting back to work, the therapist set an intention to bring it up again.

After surviving this bumpy experience of revealing her father's rage and her mother's appeasing strategies in therapy, Leonie invited her brother, Nick, to join her for a family session. She chose to ask Nick first because he had expressed concern about her flare-up of Crohn's and said he wanted to help. In session, they listened to and validated each other, and the relief of breaking the family code of silence together motivated them to continue with a recommended family therapist. The therapist noted, as did Nick, that Leonie had promptly started caretaking him after he was cast out of the family. Leonie was surprised to learn that Nick did not like her caretaking. When she fussed over him, he felt like she had no confidence in him. This activated his shaming critic, which embarrassed and angered him. After they talked it through, Nick calmed down and was less reactive with Leonie, while Leonie expressed more anger toward their parents. Nick encouraged her to take care of herself and let their parents "work out their own stuff." This idea was a challenge for Leonie's parentified part, but a breath of fresh air for other parts who felt stifled.

The Parentified Client Hands Caretaking Over to the Self of the Parent

Leonie's peacekeeper had been primed for parentification by the neglect of her developmental needs, the ongoing need of her mother's exile, and the double standard about anger. She got the message that as a girl it was her duty to take care of her mother—without resentment or anger. The protective role of parentification was reinforced with shaming and rejection whenever Leonie failed to fulfill these expectations. This legacy messaging was imparted through the family culture and down the generational line. Shamed child parts like Leonie's girl came to believe that they were unworthy of love and that their survival was in jeopardy.

Protective parts in these situations seek ways to alleviate a parent's suffering. For example, Leonie's peacekeeper, who adhered to traumatic bonds, countered the shame and pain with self-sacrifice on behalf of her negligent parents. Later, these parts transferred the traumatic bond to relationships with other people who hurt or needed her in similar ways. Much of the peacekeeper's stress was caused by perpetual caretaking and the ongoing protection of Leonie's vulnerable girl part, who carried the pain of worthlessness.

To begin the process of relieving Leonie's system of pain and fear, she and her therapist will need to unburden the caretaking legacy that promotes internal conflict between the peacekeeper and angry part. For efficiency, Leonie's therapist will unburden the legacy of parentification before seeking consent from the protectors to heal the shamed exiles who prompt their respective strategies. Because legacy burdens have been passed down from experiences of previous generations, they tend to take less time to unburden than personal burdens. Once Leonie's system is free of the legacy of parentification, her parts can more easily bond with her Self as the peacekeeper's hyper-focus on her mother becomes obsolete.

The following dialogue illustrates Leonie's process of releasing the responsibility for caring for her mother's exile back to her mother's Self. You will see the therapist engage Leonie at the start and assist with unblending the polarized protectors. Leonie notices more about these parts (e.g., thoughts, feelings, body sensations) and establishes relational connection and communication between her Self and the parts. She identifies these parts somatically and tunes into their feelings and thoughts, which segues into separation (unblending). Once Leonie's Self takes the lead, the therapist's questions become open-ended and less directive, which communicates trust in Leonie and her Self to know what is needed.

Therapist: The peacekeeping part and the angry part are both trying to help the lonely girl who feels unimportant and unloved, is that right? [*Leonie nods.*] Do you notice them in or around your body, in thoughts or feelings?

Leonie: In my head.

Therapist: How do you notice them?

> These questions help Leonie notice the parts rather than intellectualize about them. Her attention helps them unblend.

Leonie: I hear them. The peacekeeper is over here [*she touches the right side of her head*] and the angry part is over here [*she touches the left side*].

Therapist: What do you hear?

Leonie: The peacekeeper fears change, but the angry part is open.

Therapist: That's what they've been saying. Now how do you feel toward each of them?

> Checking for Self-energy

Leonie: I see they're both trying to help, so I'm grateful.

Therapist: Are they aware of your gratitude?

> Strengthening the part's relationship with the Self

Leonie: The peacekeeper is neutral, but the angry part is like "It's about time!"

Therapist: How do you respond?

Leonie: To the angry part, I say, "I'm sorry." [*Hesitates.*] But that's not me. It's the apologizer.

Leonie notices that another part has stepped in. This is new.

Therapist: Nice catch. Would the apologizing part be willing to relax? [*Leonie nods.*] What do you say to the angry part now?

Leonie: He *has* waited a long time. I know.

Therapist: Would he like your help now?

Leonie: Yes.

Therapist: Is it okay to talk with the peacekeeper now? [*Leonie nods.*] Does she feel your gratitude?

Leonie: She likes it but wants to know where this is going.

Therapist: If we help all the parts she protects, she'd be free to try something new. Would she like that?

Leonie: Sure, but she doesn't believe you can do that.

Therapist: What is she afraid would happen if she released this burden of caretaking?

Airing the protector's fears

Leonie: That's easy. No one will love me.

Therapist: Do you agree, Leonie?

Leonie: No. I don't know if my parents can love me. Maybe not. But Nick loves me, and I love him. And I've felt loved in other relationships.

Therapist: What's it like for her to hear you say that?

Asking questions that support communication between the part and Self

Leonie: She's sad. She wants my parents to love me.

Therapist: She has worked hard on that. What's she afraid would happen if she let it go?

Leonie: She'd disappear.

Therapist: No, she wouldn't. She's always going to be part of you. She'd be free to try something new. What calls to her?

Addressing the protector's fears with confidence

Leonie: She doesn't know.

Therapist: That's okay. She'll find out.

Leonie: But she needs to know my mother will be okay.

THERAPIST: She can't rescue your mother, but you can call in your mother's higher Self to help her.

Reassuring parentified parts regarding the Self of others

LEONIE: Really?

THERAPIST: Yes. As you focus inside, you can invite your mother's Self to come and help your mother.

LEONIE: [*A long pause.*] I'm seeing my mother's higher Self. She's singing in church next to my mother. But my mother has gotten small. She's a little girl now. She's watching and listening to her Self sing.

Leonie envisions her mother's Self helping her mother's exile (the little girl).

THERAPIST: How is that to see?

LEONIE: Comforting. They're holding hands. My mother likes being with her Self. They're in church. [*Leonie stops talking and starts to sway, then stops.*]

THERAPIST: How are they doing now?

LEONIE: Good. There's a hymn called "Be Thou My Vision." It's my mother's favorite Irish hymn. They were singing it together.

THERAPIST: Beautiful! Does anything else need to happen before we stop?

LEONIE: Nothing for now. That was a lot.

Legacy Unburdening

As the peacekeeper aired her fears and wishes in this session, Leonie's Self increasingly took the lead for the first time and the therapist sat back. It was a seminal moment. The realization that her mother had a Self who could help lay the groundwork for releasing the oppressive legacy that Leonie has been carrying. In the next session, the peacekeeper finally agreed to let go of her role. In IFS, this process is called *unburdening*, and it involves inviting protectors to release the weight (burden) they have been carrying. We'll talk about unburdening in more depth in the next chapter.

In Leonie's case, this process involved what IFS calls a *legacy unburdening*, meaning that this burden didn't come from her personal experience. Rather, she unconsciously picked it up from her mother. She was explicitly encouraged by her mother and others to be responsible for their feelings, and she had a part who joined with her mother out of loyalty and a desire to take some of the weight of responsibility off her mother's shoulders. In this role reversal, her childhood was much like her mother's, her grandmother's, and so on up the maternal line. Once the client's system has released a burden—either a personal burden or a legacy burden—the client can invite back qualities or feelings, like playfulness and love, that were blocked by the burden.

THERAPIST: Is the peacekeeper ready to let go of her caretaking job? [*Leonie nods.*] And she wants to invite your mother and her mother and so on to do the same, including all the women of your maternal line? [*She nods again.*] They can all let it go to light, earth, air, water, or fire. Or she may want to do it some other way.

LEONIE: Fire.

THERAPIST: When she's ready, she can invite all those women to join her with their higher Selves.

LEONIE: The men want to do it too. My father is here. He's apologizing. [*A pause.*] Nick is here too.

THERAPIST: Okay. What needs to happen?

> When the client's Self is leading, the IFS therapist should be in the role of an auxiliary witness. This very general question keeps things moving without being directional, which could interfere with the client's internal process. The therapist really has no idea what will come next.

LEONIE: We all feel sad. [*A long pause.*] My parents know they hurt us. [*Weeping*] They're so sorry.

THERAPIST: That's right. When they've all unburdened and your peacekeeper is ready, they can all go with their higher Selves.

LEONIE: They're all here. Many generations of pain. So much anger and shaming. Into the fire.

THERAPIST: Let me know when they're done.

LEONIE: [*After a long pause*] It's all in the fire.

THERAPIST: With that gone, Leonie, what do they want to invite in?

LEONIE: Kindness. Love. Joy. [*She focuses inward.*]

THERAPIST: How does that feel?

LEONIE: Great! They're hugging and singing. It's in Irish. I don't understand, but I'm feeling it.

We aim to release legacy burdens before personal burdens because the former interfere with protectors' willingness to allow access to exiles. Once Leonie's peacekeeper had released the inherited burden of parenting the adults who were supposed to be taking care of her, Leonie's protectors were willing to allow contact with the frightened girl, who had long been relegated to the outer edge of Leonie's awareness. This shift set the stage for the next step in IFS therapy—healing the exiles—which is the focus of the next chapter.

[CHAPTER 6]

IFS Health Therapy Phase 2: Healing Exiles

Exiled child parts tend to be stuck in the past, when their needs seemed like a wrong or unacceptable nuisance, which led them to believe that they were bad and unlovable. If these beliefs are not sufficiently countered by understanding, supportive adults, then the child's manager parts will reinforce them. Bolstered by criticism and anchored in shame, these painful, fear-promoting beliefs will have a negative effect on the integrated organ systems of the developing mind-body (Boyce et al., 2021). The IFS health therapy stories of Leonie, Ronan, and Tina illustrate how the Self helps exiles heal the chronic stress and suffering that follows.

In chapter 1, we introduced you to the six steps of unburdening, which we have included here again for your convenience as you read the following clinical stories. These stories illustrate the unburdening process along with adjustments you can make to adapt these steps to the needs of diverse internal systems and individual parts:

1. Unblending and witnessing
2. Rescripting
3. Retrieval
4. Unburdening ritual
5. Invitation
6. Integration

In this chapter, we'll focus on the first five steps of unburdening, while the next chapter illustrates the last step of integration. You'll notice variations in pacing, the breadth and depth of feelings, the therapist's methods of accessing parts, and more in the following examples. When the client is moving through a healing experience—either loosely or uniquely following the steps—keep going. If it's not broken, don't fix it. Your student parts will err toward being doctrinaire about the IFS blueprint. Help them relax. The client's exile decides which steps to follow and how. Parts move ahead when they're ready and go where they need to go. If you discover burdens that spontaneously release, celebrate. If exiles unexpectedly come to the present and free themselves into playfulness, don't worry about the order of the steps, just celebrate.

You can also decide to pause and focus on certain sensations, thoughts, feelings, or behaviors (like chronic hyperarousal or muscle tension) that are associated with physical problems. Revisit the explanations in this book about allostatic load, the autonomic nervous system states and parts, and known lifestyle factors affecting health. You may choose to accentuate co-regulation or the physical release of fear and tension during unburdening, or you may want to underscore the calm and courage of the Self during rescripting. Trust your intuition.

In addition, some exiles need more time and attention than others. Many are stuck in the past in unresolved, painful moments. Some want to rescue siblings; others want to know how their siblings or other family members are doing now. Before coming to the present, most exiled parts want their painful experiences witnessed and validated by the Self, while some will ask if the client's current life is an improvement over the past. Many also want to be sure the Self can provide what they needed from a caring adult in the past. The following stories provide examples of how to address all of these needs during the unburdening protocol.

Unblending and Witnessing

After protectors agree to let the client's Self connect with the exile and have unblended, the first step toward unburdening—witnessing—occurs. Here, the client's Self greets the exile, makes a repair if it asks where the Self has been, and invites the exile to show or tell its story. Recall from chapter 1 that exiles are the shamed, rejected parts who feel worthless and abandoned. Their beliefs, along with the ways in which protectors try to suppress or distract from them, are highly stressful for the body. They long to be loved and need kind, concerned, sustained attention. In this section, we illustrate the process of unblending and witnessing with Leonie (helping her work through a feeling she identified as "the void" so she could connect with her eight-year-old exile) and Ronan (helping him connect with an exile he viewed as a "bad boy").

The Void

As Leonie made various shifts and let go of inherited burdens, she allowed herself to be held with compassion by her supportive treatment team; her loving brother, Nick; her Crohn's disease peer group; and (not least!) her Self. It was a delightful new experience, but it also highlighted the lack of love and nurturing in her past. There were still times when she felt afraid and lonely, which manifested physically as the feeling of emptiness in her belly. She called this feeling *the void.* It often came with her Crohn's symptoms, but it also manifested in seemingly random moments. Here is her inquiry into the void.

Therapist: You're feeling the void right now? [*Leonie nods.*] Ready to find out what's going on? [*She nods again.*] Focus on it. What do you notice?

Focusing on the physical feeling of emptiness to find the part who's feeling it

Leonie: It's emptiness, but, at the same time, pain . . . I can't find words . . . Or maybe too many words apply.

Therapist: How do you feel toward it?

Leonie: Scared . . . No, *it's* scared. This is the eight-year-old. I want to back up. This feeling creeps up on me, and when I notice it, I feel overwhelmed.

Given that Leonie was struggling to connect with this young part, the therapist opted for the *room technique*, a type of containment imagery for increasing safety with potentially challenging parts. This technique involves imagining putting the part in a safe room, separate at first from the client's Self and other parts, who are all outside the room. This calms protectors who fear that the target part will unblend and be out of control in some way, which helps them unblend from the client's Self. Once the client feels curious and caring toward the target part, other parts are usually willing to let the client's Self go into the room with the target part for a conversation. During this next dialogue, you'll see an angry part come out to express what the target part could not express at the time.

Therapist: Let's put her in a room. A nice, comfortable room. And for now, you be outside the room with all your other parts.

Leonie: Okay.

Therapist: Is she there?

Leonie: Yes.

Therapist: How do you feel toward her?

Leonie: So sad! Something's wrong.

Therapist: What is it?

Leonie: Oh! She's in her room and she hears my father beating Nick. He's swearing and Nick is yelling something, and she hears a thud and knows Nick got thrown at the wall.

Therapist: Oh, Leonie! How awful.

Leonie's Angry Part: [*Opens her eyes, sits straighter, and balls a fist.*] I want to get that baseball bat and beat him to death!

An angry part blends.

Therapist: Of course you wanted to do that. But Leonie was too little to protect her brother, wasn't she?

The therapist speaks to the angry part directly, without calling on Leonie's Self to be in the middle.

Leonie's Angry Part: I could have stabbed him in his sleep.

The angry part of the little girl comes out to express outrage.

Therapist: Are you there, Leonie?

The therapist checks to see if Leonie's Self is available.

Leonie: [*After a few beats*] Yes. But that angry part of her still wants to kill their father.

Therapist: Do her feelings make sense to you?

Leonie: Yes!

Therapist: Who wouldn't be angry? It's okay that she wants to kill him. Let her know you understand.

Leonie: She's relieved that I get it. [*A long pause with changes in facial expression.*] She just showed me what she wants to do to him.

Therapist: How was that for her?

Leonie: Good! And weirdly fine for me too. I understand. She's carried this outrage for too long.

Therapist: Is she aware that Nick is alive and grown up? [*She shakes her head.*] Let her know that Nick lives near you. You're both grown up. He's okay now. [*A long pause.*] If the angry part will let us help the girl, we can get everyone out of the past. They could all come live with you and Nick in the present. Would that be good?

Updating a part who is stuck in the past

Therapist: Is she willing to let us help the girl? [*Leonie nods.*] Is she there? [*Leonie nods again.*] How do you feel toward the girl?

Leonie: I want to help.

Therapist: What does she need?

Leonie: She wants me to know what happened and to get her out of there.

Therapist: Is there more she needs you to know?

Leonie: Just how scary it was and how helpless she felt.

Therapist: Does she want to come to the present?

Leonie: Yes. She wants me to get Nick, too, but she wonders if I can.

Therapist: Sure you can. Your father has a higher Self always ready to help, but it's up to him to accept that help. He's not their problem anymore. You can take care of anything she wants you to. You can even pause him in that scene just like you pause a video so Nick and the little girl can leave with you safely. Whatever works for her.

Leonie: She likes that idea.

The therapist uses a *pause button* to help Leonie solve a challenge in the scene.

Therapist: Let me know when it's done. [*Leonie nods.*] Are they ready to leave now? [*Leonie nods again.*] Does the little girl want to come to the present or go to a fantasy place?

Leonie: The present.

Therapist: How are she and Nick doing now?

Leonie: Good.

Therapist: What did that experience with her father make the little girl feel about herself?

Leonie: Spineless, bad, sinful. It helped to let the angry part express the outrage.

Therapist: How do you feel toward her now?

Leonie: I love her.

Therapist: Is she ready to let go of those false beliefs about who she is?

Leonie: She is.

In this session, Leonie watched herself as an eight-year-old girl listening helplessly as her father assaulted her brother. As the girl conveyed her profound sadness, fear, and impotence, a homicidal young part interrupted. After speaking with it directly, the therapist brought Leonie's Self back in. With her Self as a witness, the angry part expressed the outrage it had never been able to reveal. This gave Leonie's system a chance to see that the forbidden feeling and fantasy were benign when witnessed with compassion inside. Afterward, the therapist and Leonie negotiated to have her Self help the girl. As soon as Leonie's Self had witnessed this event, the angry part felt relieved, and when the girl knew that Nick was now okay, she was ready to leave the past.

However, after feeling the possibility and promise of unburdening, Leonie experienced grief over the loss of time. Her peacekeeper said this after the girl unburdened: "I spent so much time trying to keep things that I can't control under control! I wasted so much time." Grief, which is common after unburdenings, needs time and space.

Therapist: I hear the grief, Leonie. Is that the girl who tried hard to keep the peace in the family? [*Leonie nods.*] Do you understand how she feels?

Leonie: I do! She poured a lot of energy into trying to make the family safer.

Therapist: Let her know you get that. See if she can take in your understanding.

Leonie: She is.

Therapist: Does she need anything?

Leonie: Just the time and space to feel what she feels that's happening right now. Not having to pretend.

Therapist: Stay with her.

Leonie: I am.

Therapist: You really are.

Leonie set an intention to follow up with the grieving part; the girl who felt terrified, helpless, and alone; her angry protector; and other parts who needed more time, attention, and support to be ready to transition to new roles.

A Bad Boy

When Ronan was seven years old, he would walk home after school every day wondering where the bully would be waiting. Since there were no grown-ups in sight or waiting at home, and his older brother was at soccer practice, Ronan was always on his own. After catching him, the bully would hit, spit on, and choke Ronan. Since the bully was bigger, this abuse went on for years until Ronan got big enough to fight back. During those years, Ronan struggled to focus and learn in school, and the adults, incurious and ignorant of his trauma, blamed him. Although Ronan felt loved by his mother and, later, by his ineffectual but kind stepfather, he longed for people to see the good in him, validate his perspective, understand his feelings, and help him instead of viewing him as a "bad boy." That was the promise of therapy.

At the start of the following session, Ronan and his therapist reviewed his parts map (see page 67) to remember where the last session had ended. Since then, Ronan had shown up for his protectors and gained some trust, which had lowered the temperature on their polarizations. In the following dialogue, Ronan gets permission from the protectors to proceed with this exiled child and Ronan's Self goes back in time—as a trustworthy, available adult—to rescue him.

RONAN: My neck and shoulders are all knotted, and I feel sick to my stomach.

THERAPIST: That's a lot of physical tension. What else do you notice?

Guiding Ronan to find the part

RONAN: It's the boy. He needs to move. He feels trapped in school. He can't sit still, but he's afraid of getting in trouble. The more he moves, the more afraid he feels and the more he needs to move.

THERAPIST: How do you feel toward him?

Checking for Self-energy

RONAN: I care about him, but I wish he'd relax and quit getting in trouble!

Ronan speaks from another part.

THERAPIST: So, another part wants him to relax. Would it be willing to let the capable, grown-up you handle this?

Asking the part to unblend

RONAN: Okay. It's cautious but willing to give me some space. [*His shoulders drop as he exhales.*]

THERAPIST: That was a good, deep breath. How do you feel toward the boy now?

Checking again for Self-energy

RONAN: I care, but the teacher is eyeing him. She has an attitude. He sees that, too, and it scares him. I know what's coming. I have a rageful part that wants to say something to her.

THERAPIST: What does it want to say to her?

RONAN: He's a teenager. He's swearing.

THERAPIST: He's mad, I get that, but if he were to say something substantial to her, what would it be?

RONAN: He'd say, "Grown-ups who pick on little kids are disgusting and weak. That's what you are."

THERAPIST: Would he like to say that to her? [*Ronan nods.*] Does he want you to say it, or does he want to say it?

RONAN: He wants to.

Rescripting

In this next part of the dialogue, Ronan takes the second step toward unburdening—rescripting (or a "do-over")—in which the client's Self offers to come back in time and provide whatever the exile needed in that moment. More generally, this step prompts the exile to take charge and direct the action of the do-over toward a desirable outcome.

THERAPIST: One thing first. Let's call in this teacher's higher Self to take her away afterward and help her learn. That way none of your parts will need to think about her again. Okay?

> Releasing the angry part and increasing safety

RONAN: He likes that.

THERAPIST: Let me know when this angry teenage part is done speaking to the teacher. [*Ronan nods.*] How's the boy doing now?

RONAN: The boy is still trying to sit still. He doesn't see me.

THERAPIST: What needs to happen?

> Here is that nondirective question again, which the therapist uses when the client has sufficient Self-energy to lead.

RONAN: I'm telling the boy that she's gone.

THERAPIST: He didn't notice her leave. Show him that she's gone now and that the teenager stood up for him.

> Reinforcing safety and developing a positive exile-protector relationship

RONAN: But the boy wants to say something too.

THERAPIST: Sure. He can do that. We can bring her back or—

RONAN: No! He'll send a messenger.

THERAPIST: What does he want to say?

RONAN: He wants the messenger to say, "I'm a nice person! Don't be mean."

THERAPIST: How does that feel?

Ronan: Good. I'm telling the boy that some kids need to move a lot and it's okay. But he feels anxious all the time and that's not so good.

Therapist: Would he like your help with that?

Building trust in the Self-to-part relationship

Ronan: Yes.

Therapist: To help him, where should we go first?

Ronan: He wants a hug first. Then he wants me to walk him home from school. He has things to show me.

As Ronan's Self and the boy walked home, the boy asked why Ronan hadn't come sooner. Ronan thought about this and answered that he got crowded out by everyone's fear. The boy said he was still afraid and Ronan replied, "I know. I can feel it." The boy was surprised that anyone would bother with his feelings. Ronan said it wasn't a bother, and the boy asked if Ronan would stick around. Ronan said yes.

They continued walking together and found the bully was hiding behind a tree. Ronan's Self explained to both of them that the abuse would never happen again and invited the boy to tell the bully what it had been like for him; then they sent the bully off with his higher Self. After that, they proceeded to the boy's empty house and discussed what to do. The boy wanted to leave but didn't want to abandon his mother. Ronan suggested having her meet and marry his stepfather right away so she wouldn't be alone. Here is the conclusion to their conversation.

Ronan: Yes! He likes that. He wants her to be happy.

Therapist: What needs to happen?

Ronan: He'll invite my stepfather back to that time so they can meet right away. Everyone likes that.

Retrieval and Unburdening Ritual

With this resolution, the boy was ready to leave the past with Ronan and come to live in the present, which represents the third step of unburdening—retrieval. Once the boy felt grounded in the present, he was ready for the fourth step—unburdening, a ritual in which the client releases the burden, often to one of the five elements (light, earth, air, water, fire). For example, the part may choose to send the burden off with bright light, bury it, throw it to the wind, release it in the ocean, or burn it in a bonfire. In contrast, some people devise a more personal way of letting their burdens go. It's up to them. Here is how Ronan's boy released the traumatic beliefs and stuck feelings that were trapping him.

Therapist: Is he ready to come to the present with you now and unload those burdens?

Ronan: He's ready! [*A pause.*] He wants to go to the jobsite with me.

Therapist: To unload burdens? [*Ronan nods.*] I bet he wants to bury them. Am I right?

Ronan: Totally! [*They laugh.*] We're digging a giant hole with the excavator.

THERAPIST: Perfect. Now what?

RONAN: We're at the edge of the hole. There's a pile of stuff that looks like big, dark boulders. We're dropping them in with the excavator one by one. There's this deep thud when they hit the earth at the bottom of the hole. [*A pause.*] Now we're piling dirt on top.

THERAPIST: How is that for him?

RONAN: Thrilling!

THERAPIST: Let me know when it's done.

RONAN: [*A long pause.*] Yep. It's buried. There's a big open space on top.

THERAPIST: [*Another long pause.*] How does that feel?

RONAN: Great.

Invitation

At this point in the dialogue, Ronan was moving into the fifth step of unburdening—the invitation—in which the exile invites the qualities he needs and wants going forward into his mind and body. Some parts visualize the process of taking in the desirable qualities; others have a tactile experience. Some people name the qualities aloud, as you'll see with Ronan's exile.

THERAPIST: What qualities would he like to invite in that will help him going forward?

RONAN: Play. We're building a playground on top of the dirt. It's fantastic. He's running around trying everything.

Ronan's boy embodies play.

THERAPIST: Great. What else?

RONAN: Freedom.

THERAPIST: How does that feel?

RONAN: Without the weight of the world on him, he feels lighter. He's a happy kid. He has fun.

THERAPIST: Anything else?

RONAN: He wants me to know that he's a good person . . . I know that. He said he wants to be loved, and I said, "I love you."

THERAPIST: How did that feel?

RONAN: [*Breathing deeply*] It was a big relief.

THERAPIST: [*Breathing with Ronan*] Hmm . . . Let that relief sink in.

In this session, the boy was able to come to the present and let go of the notion that he was bad and deserved to be in pain. Over the next weeks in therapy, Ronan returned to various other challenging events and situations to collect some even younger parts. Along the way, he noticed and gave thanks for the cleverness and resilience of his protectors. He explained, "They see me and they're not so afraid anymore. They like their story having a new ending. I tell them how brave and smart they were to get through all those bad things. Well, I don't *tell* them because we don't need words. I feel it toward them, and they feel me and know it's true."

Experiential Exercise: A Post-Unburdening Body Scan

You can do the following optional post-unburdening body scan to consolidate the experience of releasing burdens in mind and body. You can do this in session with a client, with the option of creating a recording for them to take home. Some clients like to listen to it again at home as a guided meditation. Go slowly—slower than seems necessary—pausing throughout to allow time to reflect and notice inside.

Notice what it's like to exhale that [*name the burden*]... to feel the space... to feel that relief.

[*Pause*]

In your chest... neck... shoulders... and jaw... That's the connection with your Self inside.

[Pause]

Now, starting at the top of your head and going all the way down to your stomach [*slowly add other areas of significance, pausing in between*], notice how the relief shows up.

[Pause]

How does it affect your parts?

[Pause]

If they'd like to, they can lean into you... feel you here... feel your concern and care.

[Pause]

Now you can take a physical imprint of this physical state as you breathe together and exhale into even deeper calm... more relaxation... greater connection... and that deep relief.

A Baby Part Unburdens

Although parts can be nonverbal, baby parts are preverbal. When a baby unburdens, the healing steps are typically sensory. Like any baby, an exiled baby part needs attention and holding. As the client attunes to the baby's emotional and physical experience, emotionally charged images may arise, some of which may seem to be metaphoric. For example, the client may see the baby as blue, and other parts may insist that it is dead. Or the client may see or feel the baby part being stuck at the bottom of a well or in a dark, cold cave.

Alternatively, the images may be literal. For instance, the baby may be alone in a crib with a dirty diaper or may be being physically or sexually abused. Some clients are haunted by these kinds of images but dismiss them as bizarre and untrue. We advise against interpreting them or ignoring them. Instead, check for reactive parts and then let the client's Self rescue the baby. Sometimes, older parts—from toddlerhood up—draw the client's attention to a baby part. Ultimately, these young protectors need attention too. Remind the client to relieve them of their caretaking roles and discuss their developmental needs. (See appendix C.)

To illustrate this phenomenon, let's return to Tina, the client with metabolic syndrome who entered treatment with concerns about developing type 2 diabetes and cardiovascular disease. So far, Tina's therapist had helped her notice a team of anxious, hardworking managers who were in charge all day—keeping her on top of work, parenting, and running a household. Once her kids were in bed, a team of firefighters took over, guiding her to watch TV to numb her mind, self-soothe with snacks, and stay up late in a dissociative state of escape. The last dialogue with Tina ended as she was getting in touch with a sad part who felt dread related to existential fears of death, and then felt both relief and frustration when a spacey, dissociative part stepped in to stop the feelings.

The therapist and Tina had agreed to get permission from any protector with concerns before returning to the trailhead of sadness and dread, which you will see as they continue their work. In the following dialogue, Tina and her therapist begin with the snacking part and opt for explicit direct access as a method of gaining understanding and eventually unblending. Tina holds Self-energy while consciously being in the snacking part's mind-body experience. You'll see Tina and the therapist unblend several protectors and gain consent to connect with the sad exile in a relational healing process. The dialogue begins with the snacker in front of the freezer looking for ice cream.

Therapist: How do you feel toward the snacker?

Tina: I'm curious and want to help it. [*Pauses.*] I really want to know what it is about ice cream that is more important than my health.

> Note that Tina's inner critic chimes in right after she says she's curious.

Therapist: Can the critic relax and allow the you who is curious to do the helping?

> Now that Tina is well aware of her parts, the therapist can just speak to what they have both noticed and ask the critical part to step back and unblend.

Tina: Yeah, it stepped in for just a moment. It's gone now. [*Pauses.*] I feel urgency. [*Pauses again.*] Now I'm sitting down in front of the TV with a bowl of ice cream and the feeling is like, *Phew!*

Therapist: You're seeing through the eyes of the snacker now? [*Tina nods.*] Is it willing to open some space for you?

Tina: When I ask, the connection goes. [*Pauses.*] It's easier for me to *be* the snacker.

Therapist: Okay. The snacker can blend and you can still be there. How open and interested do you feel toward it?

Tina: Very. [*Pauses.*] I want to know what it's like for this part.

Therapist: [*Nods.*] I'm going to talk to the snacker directly and you can listen. Okay? [*Tina nods.*] Are you there?

> Transitioning to explicit direct access

Tina's Snacker Part: I just want to enjoy the ice cream. I don't want anyone to bother me. It's so soothing, cool, and creamy. I love everything about it.

Therapist: What would happen if you stopped eating ice cream?

Tina's Snacker Part: She'll want to fix everything for everyone, and she'll get exhausted, but she'll push through until she burns out. And from there it'll get worse. [*Pauses.*] That feeling of dread that she gets sometimes? That's the tip of the iceberg.

Therapist: A powerful motive! Tina, are you there listening? [*Tina nods.*] Do you know what the snacker is talking about?

Tina: I know burnout. I know that feeling of dread. I avoid it if I can.

Therapist: What do you say to this part?

Tina: I get it about snacking. It's a relief! Especially when I'm stressed. The snacker helps me forget the dread.

Therapist: Does it feel your appreciation? [*Tina nods.*] Is it willing to let you help the part or parts who dread something?

Tina: [*Shrugs.*] It's like, "Suit yourself!" [*After a long pause, her expression gradually changes.*]

Therapist: What's happening?

Tina: [*In a strained voice*] I feel anxiety . . . and dread.

Therapist: What do you hear?

Tina: It's like, "Don't feel that!"

A protector who wards off the anxious part reveals itself.

Therapist: Would that part let you help the anxious one? [*After a pause, Tina nods.*] How do you feel toward the anxious part now?

Tina: I want to help it. Will it let me?

Therapist: Invite it to open some breathing room for you. [*Pauses.*] That's right. Slowly breathing together. Yes, just like that.

Breathing to reduce panic and hyperarousal

Tina: [*Inhaling and exhaling slowly with her eyes closed*] Better.

Therapist: Let it know you're here to help.

Tina: It's relieved.

Therapist: How old is it?

Tina: Young.

Therapist: What does it need?

Inviting the part to speak for its needs

Tina: She wants to sit on my lap in a big bean bag chair with a fuzzy blanket. And our cat, Nimby. It's her safe nest.

> Note that Tina switches to the pronoun *she*.

Therapist: Perfect. Does she protect anyone else?

Tina: The part who feels dread.

Therapist: Will she let you help that part?

> Relieving a young manager of responsibility

Tina: She's okay with that as long as she and Nimby can stay nearby.

Therapist: Great. Is it okay to pay attention to the dread now?

> Asking permission to go to the exile

Tina: Yes. [*Tina starts making a small, subtle rocking motion.*]

Therapist: Let me know what's happening if you need support.

Tina: My belly feels hollow. [*She starts panting.*] It's dark. I'm alone. I feel dread and despair. [*She starts to cry and rock.*]

Therapist: Are you there with this part, Tina?

> The therapist checks on Tina's ability to stay with the part and witness it from Self. Although Tina's feelings are clearly intense, she doesn't seem anxious.

Tina: [*Wrapping her arms around her body*] I'm with her.

Therapist: Great. [*After a few beats, as Tina moans sorrowfully*] That's right. Let the feelings come in waves and recede. [*Pauses for a few beats.*] Hmm . . . Be there with her in just the way she needs.

> Reading cues and soothing vocally with "That's right," the therapist makes some soothing sounds like *hmm* to acknowledge she's witnessing and present with the process.

Tina: [*Covers her face and wails. After a few minutes, the crying slows, then stops, then restarts, and so on. Finally, she shudders, inhales deeply, stops crying, and opens her eyes.*]

Tina: She's a baby. It's cold and damp. I'm warming her with my body.

Therapist: Babies are small. Does she feel how big and warm you are? [*Tina nods.*] Notice the warmth your bodies are sharing, the softness, the comfort. [*Pauses.*] Notice from both perspectives—yours of holding and hers of being held. How does that feel? [*Tina nods calmly.*] You can notice her needs and simply meet them.

> Enhancing the therapeutic relationship between the Self and the exile

Tina: [*After a long pause*] Now she's warm and dry.

Therapist: Wonderful! [*Tina continues to rock gently.*] Take a physical imprint of this moment. You're holding her; she's being held. You're rocking her; she's feeling warm and steady. You can come back to this anytime. [*Pauses.*] Is it okay for the girl who gets sad and anxious and the cat Nimby to see the baby now?

Making sure that the young manager is updated and feels included

Tina: She's here. We're all in the nest together.

Therapist: Are the snacker and fixer parts aware of what just happened?

Prompting Tina's Self to update the other protectors about the unburdening of the baby exile, a significant change for them too

Tina: They weren't, but now they are!

At the start of this session, Tina's critical fixer part agreed that she could interview the snacker—a reactive protector who was in the habit of jumping in to suppress the baby exile's existential hunger and despair with comfort food. Tina needed to befriend the snacker and get its permission to rescue the baby exile. After the baby unburdened, Tina invited the fixer and snacker to see her Self taking care of the baby, which helped them trust her and encouraged them to consider what they'd like to do if they could leave their extreme roles. As polarized protectors calm down, the whole internal system gets more access to the Self and can digest the news that everyone is welcome and loved. Before the end of the session, Tina took time to absorb the "imprint" of being with the baby, now warm and safe, and set an intention to check in with the baby during two predictably recurring moments in her day: her morning wake-up ritual and at red-light stops on the way home from work.

After finding the baby part, Tina wondered if her mother had suffered from postpartum depression. Sure enough, Tina found out that her mother had been depressed for several months in the first year of Tina's life. She also learned that her mother had suffered gestational diabetes during pregnancy, a condition associated with epigenetic changes that increased the risk of metabolic syndrome for both Tina and her mother later in life (Al Bekai et al., 2025; Xiang, 2023). This piece of information gave Tina's parts a more nuanced view of her disease, which was the result of a complex combination of factors. "It's not about fault or shamefulness," she concluded.

As Tina's vignette illustrates, once an exile unburdens and protectors are aware or updated, protectors who have been in conflict (like Tina's fixer and snacker) have the opportunity to reconcile. Sometimes, when protective parts are aware of what's unfolding, this happens spontaneously during the unburdening. If not, we can facilitate a repair by checking in with them and asking if they still need to fear each other. Aside from settling protector conflicts, we ask protectors if they are ready to (1) retire from extreme roles, and (2) choose a new role according to their interests. After an unburdening, as well as periodically throughout treatment, the therapist and client review beneficial shifts.

Dissociative Protectors

For Tina—as for many clients with dissociative, "spacey" parts—the nonverbal unburdening of an infant part can feel dreamlike and fade out of consciousness once the client returns to their day-to-day life. If this is not addressed, it can derail the post-unburdening integration process. To address this risk, Tina updated her parts map, a visual reminder to self-reflect and follow up. As you can see in this updated map, Tina chose to add the baby and the baby's protectors, as well as all the significant parts she had noticed at this point in therapy, including the sad little girl who had previously emerged.

Tina's Parts Map, Version 3

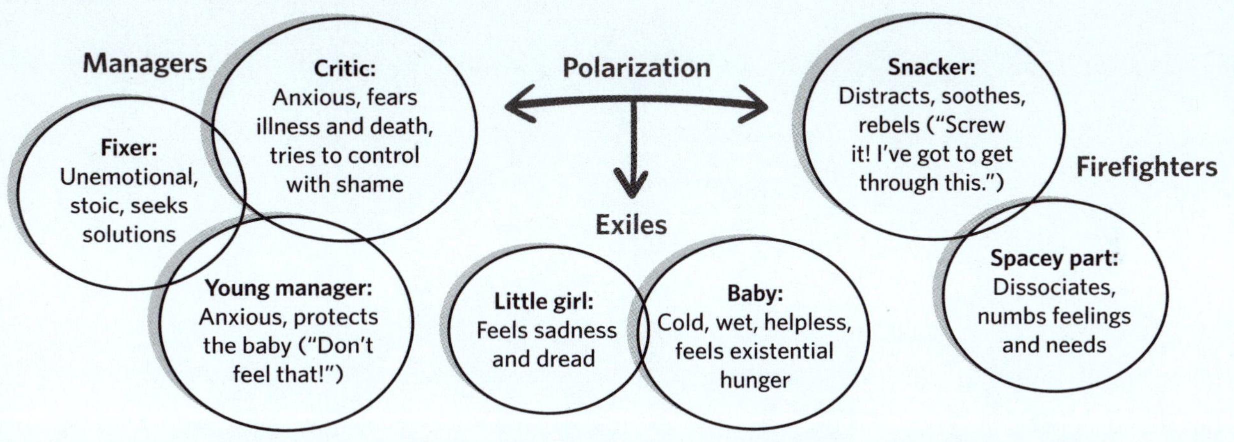

After the session, Tina described physically co-regulating with the baby, a process that reduced the baby's hyperarousal and dysregulation. She also described her experience prior to unburdening this exile: "Before being held and holding the baby like this, I felt trapped and stranded in a dark place beyond hope. It seemed I would die there alone. Maybe I wanted to die rather than live not knowing if it would ever end. Whenever I'm alone, that feeling comes up. That's when I usually run to the freezer for ice cream. Now I come back to the warmth of holding the baby, and the baby feeling the warmth of being held. It's a physical safety that calms both of us. I can feel it right now as I describe it." Would this practice contribute to reductions in her insulin resistance? We had to keep going to find out. ▍

[CHAPTER 7]

IFS Health Therapy Phase 3: Integration and a Balanced Life

When our exiles release burdens, they start forward on a new path with Self-energy flowing around the body. Although they no longer have to contend with the shame, fear, and unmet needs that they've released, protectors can still hold on to lifelong protective strategies after unburdening. While the previous unburdening steps heal the pain that drives protector tactics, *integration* frees them from burden-driven thinking, speaking, and behavior that lands heavily on our relationships and health. The IFS health therapy integration process maximizes regulation and the physiological and emotional relief of the unburdened internal social system. Now, protectors who contribute to the client's health risk (like Tina's snacking part, Ronan's rageful part, and Leonie's peacekeeper) can consider:

- Am I ready to stop doing this job? Fully or partially?
- If not, what needs to change so that I can stop?
- What calls to me going forward?
- What would it feel like and look like to have my Self available to me in my relationships with family and friends, at work, in school, and elsewhere in my community?
- How do I feel about my body now? How will I take care of it?
- How do I feel about other parts? What do I want from other people? From my Self?
- What protective habits do I still slide into that don't serve my health and well-being? Am I ready to change these habits?

During integration, the Self (1) checks in with all the protectors related to the illness to be sure they are aware of the unburdening and updates any parts who were not watching, (2) reinforces the exile's healing with regular Self-to-part contact, (3) deepens connection with protectors and facilitates understanding and rapprochement between parts who have been in conflict, (4) asks protectors what interests them and if they're ready to retire, (5) supports change from burden-driven roles and chronic stress to the development of Self-led pursuits and relationships, including with the body to support healing, and (6) reviews beneficial shifts in the system.

In the session following Tina's baby unburdening, the therapist checked in with her to find out how the baby was doing. After an unburdening, we facilitate integration by helping clients foster regular contact with the exile, thus maintaining the flow of energy between their exile and Self. Tina continued this practice until the relational safety between her exile and Self felt secure. She used the *physical imprint* technique (Sowell, 2024)—which is a somatic, relational cue for returning to and strengthening the calm connection between a part and the Self—as illustrated in the baby's unburdening in chapter 6. Here is Tina's description of her post-unburdening integration process with the baby:

> "I tune in to the baby when I wake up in the morning before I jump out of bed. I put my hand right over my heart and go back to the physical imprint of holding her. Sometimes I hang out there for a while and sometimes it's just a moment, but it's relaxing for both of us. I also check in later in the day on my way home from work. There's a row of stoplights. When they're red, I take a moment and go back to the warmth and safety in my body of holding her. It's surprising how just seconds of being together feels calming and deepens our connection. She's more relaxed and so am I—all the time, not just when I'm with her."

Experiential Exercise: Physical Imprinting

This practice is designed to help clients anchor and recall an embodied experience of Self-energy. It can be used after a moment of connection with Self, such as an experience of awe, a sense of oneness with nature, or any moment that evoked a strong feeling of presence in the body. To begin, invite the client to recall a moment when they felt connected to Self in the body. Then invite them to take some time to capture this moment using the following script:

1. Feel yourself in that moment. Where are you? What do you see? Are you doing anything or simply being?
2. Tune into the physical experience. Notice how the sensations in your body begin to unfold.
3. Feel the connection with your Self. Feel the energy as it flows through you and your body, radiating from the center of your chest.
4. Notice whatever sensations arise. Maybe you notice a sense of awe or lightness filling you. Just take some time to notice whatever stands out. There is no need to think. Just be in the moment with the flow of connectedness in your body.
5. As you stay with these sensations, feel the energy in your chest extending out in all directions:
    - Down to your belly and gut
    - Up into your neck, head, and face
    - Out into your shoulders
    - Into your arms, hands, and fingers
    - Spreading through your upper back and all the way down to your lower back
    - Into your hips and the base of your torso
    - Down through your legs and all the way into your feet and toes
6. As you focus on the most powerful sensations of Self in the body, take a physical imprint of the experience. This imprint will become a somatic memory—a body-based cue for coming back to Self in the body.
7. As you go forward, use this practice in moments when you already feel some safety. Once that is easy enough, try using it during more challenging situations to return to Self in the body.

When protectors are no longer tasked with keeping emotional pain out of mind, they can relax. Young managers like Tina's anxious part can make requests and play. Older protectors can collaborate across complementary areas of interest. For example, some may choose to specialize in building relationships with healthy boundaries or deepening existing bonds, while others may choose to take up new pursuits like music or art. Still others may focus on supporting the needs of their mind-body—by relaxing more, meditating, or transforming old habits—or attend to practical matters like navigating job responsibilities, managing finances, or making needed changes at home or in work. Others may look to the spiritual realms for more healing, direction, and meaning. While exiles like Tina's baby part can still feel hurt when a painful external event occurs, present-day incidents no longer land on unhealed wounds. The availability of the Self makes all the difference.

As Tina described her integration practice with the baby, she felt calmer. The therapist drew attention to this for the benefit of her protectors, aiming to bolster their awareness of and trust in Tina's Self, and to offer them the possibility of deepening connection and calm in the body via the Self-to-part relationship. In the following dialogue, Tina remains focused inward, while the therapist observes and highlights Tina's physical relaxation to support future reconnection with her protectors.

THERAPIST: Are you feeling that calm connection as you're describing this practice with the baby? [*Tina nods.*] Can you check with the exile's team of protectors [*the young, anxious manager; the fixer; the critic; the snacking part; and the spacey one*] and invite them to notice you and this deepening relaxation in your body?

TINA: They feel calm with me and in my body. It's very noticeable.

THERAPIST: What do you notice?

TINA: They feel relaxed, and so does my body, especially in my upper body—my shoulders and neck. I feel warmer, and the tension in my belly is gone.

> The therapist observes Tina's physical relaxation, her calmness, and the slow rise and fall of her chest as she breathes, highlighting these cues for Tina's parts.

THERAPIST: As you're feeling calm and peaceful inside together, notice the warmth and relaxation in your face, neck, and shoulders—down into your chest and stomach. Now stay with that and invite everyone to take a physical imprint of this calm connection so you can return to it with your protectors in the future. [*Tina nods and wraps her arms around herself.*] Let me know when that's complete.

TINA: We've got it.

THERAPIST: Is there anything else you want to communicate to them?

TINA: Yes, but I'm not totally sure how.

THERAPIST: You've been doing great going inside and communicating with them in words but also through the body. [*Tina nods.*] Can the part that's not sure relax and trust *you* to know?

TINA: Yeah, it's okay. I've got this. [*Tina goes inside for several minutes.*] They totally felt that.

Therapist: What did they feel?

Tina: The calm, but also how much I want to keep progressing and get well. And that I appreciate them and want to help them be free to do whatever they want.

Therapist: Beautiful, Tina. How did you communicate that to them?

Tina: I focused on my heart like I do with the baby and held the group of them in my mind. Once I felt the connection with them, I focused on my gratitude and how much I want them to be free.

In this dialogue, you saw an example of integration with the baby exile's team of protectors. Tina described how she was following up with the baby post-unburdening through a daily practice of co-regulation, using the physical imprint of calm and safety in her body as a doorway to secure connection with her Self. She then turned her attention to her protectors to increase relaxation throughout her mind-body. With support from her therapist, Tina realized that her self-doubt was a part she could unblend, which gave her the reassuring experience of feeling her Self come online through a mind-body connection with her protectors.

In connection with her Self, Tina described her parts feeling more security and compassion inside, which can contribute to the emotional and autonomic regulation that supports health (Luo et al., 2018). The Self-to-part relationship serves as a stepping stone from which to build unblending skills in increasingly challenging situations, when parts are faced with moments that test their capacity to hold Self-energy and return to regulation. By modeling confidence in Tina's ability to unblend and access her Self, the therapist reinforced Tina's trust in her own capacity to regulate and lead her parts. Clients' confidence increases as they repeatedly experience the power of unblending and the availability of Self-energy. For Tina, her confidence was growing alongside her ability to return to calm as she became more aware of her parts and her ability to access Self.

Experiential Exercise: Self-Love and Compassion Meditation

So many people believe that loving themselves and taking care of their own needs is selfish. They are taught, directly or indirectly, that being a virtuous person is all about loving others, serving others, or even giving to others what parts of us still need. Sometimes, this belief comes from hardworking, well-intended protector parts who stepped in when more vulnerable exiles didn't get the love and attention they needed. The following meditation is dedicated to these vulnerable parts who needed more care, as well as to the protective parts that have worked so hard on their behalf. As clients move through this exercise, invite them to notice whatever parts come forward and bring gentle curiosity to them.

- Take a moment to settle into the space inside . . . noticing the thoughts, body sensations, and other signs of your parts doing all that they do on your behalf . . . always feeling something, thinking something, responding, working so hard at your life.
- As you hold your awareness of them now—as you notice their thoughts, emotions, or physical sensations moving through you—allow yourself to realize their devotion . . . how much responsibility they carry . . . how alone they have been at times.
- As you become aware of them, see if it's possible to send them love and appreciation.
- Invite them to notice your presence as you direct your Self-energy to them, maybe breathing your love and appreciation to them . . . maybe saying: "I feel you. I'm listening to you. I love you." Invite them into this heart-space with you . . . to really feel your love and appreciation, maybe as warmth or light or something else that helps them. Invite them to lean into it . . . into your Self-energy . . . and take it in. Invite them to bask in it . . . breathe it in . . . absorb it like warm sunlight or clean fresh air.
- Invite them to take a physical imprint of this connection in the body with your Self—the warmth, the ease of breathing, the energy of the heart.
- If you have parts that are opposed to this idea, see if they would be willing to relax back just for a few minutes and see if it's all right to do this. If not, that's okay. They may need you to listen to their thoughts and concerns and stay with them right now.
- Staying with this process, see if there is anything that they need or would like from you going forward . . . Invite them to communicate that to you now. If it feels right, set an intention with them, something realistic and doable.

Circling Back to Go Forward

As Tina and her therapist checked in with the protectors after the baby's unburdening to see who was ready to change their role, Tina heard a clear "no" from the snacking part, a key player in Tina's goal of healing change. "When I ask it why, it says, 'It would be too sad.'" This response pointed to a burdened exile, a sad little girl who came up briefly in one of Tina's early sessions (see page 74). With the recognition of another part in need of unburdening, the IFS healing process can circle back to unblending and unburdening. We flexibly rotate between unblending, unburdening, and integration whenever necessary as different parts and their needs surface. The sad girl, who Tina dubbed *Little Tina*, needed to be unburdened to continue the healing process.

With her therapist's support and Self-energy available inside, Tina returned to the 6 F's and the steps of unburdening. She witnessed scenes from Little Tina's life after her father's immigration to the United States: "She doesn't know when she'll see her father again. It's like someone died. There's a lonely feeling in the house. Her father's chair at the table is empty. She feels a hollow pit in her belly. It's a bad feeling when she wakes up and goes to sleep at night." With her Self leading the way, Tina went back in time and rescued Little Tina.

Once Tina helped this little girl release the sadness, dread, and other burdens, she felt a deep feeling of relief in her body. Tina returned to her protective system to ensure they were aware of this change and to see if anyone was ready to unload their extreme role. The anxious young protector immediately stepped forward, releasing her anxiety into warm sunlight. Afterward, she wanted to run and play with Little Tina at their favorite playground. As Tina visualized her young protector and unburdened exile playing, she remembered the power and joy of playing on swings during happier times in her childhood—the feeling of leaning back, pumping her legs, and reaching her feet toward the sky.

In the next session, Tina reported a significant shift: One day, when she took her children to the park, she spontaneously joined them on the swings, guided by the joy, safety, and trust she felt inside. Joining her children on the swings was exactly what she needed to feel more balance and well-being in her body. Indeed, the rhythmic activities that children naturally gravitate toward—such as swinging, jumping on a trampoline, swaying, dancing, or skipping rope—stimulate the balance centers of the inner ear (the vestibular system) and the nucleus tractus solitarius, which is a key brainstem center that plays a role in sensory integration and autonomic regulation. These sensory and vestibular inputs help calm and organize the nervous system by promoting parasympathetic balance and improving vagal tone and heart rate variability, which translates to resilience and well-being. With our parts unburdened and the presence of Self in the body, our natural healing inclinations to play and socially connect can emerge.

Natural Vagus Nerve–Stimulating Activities

Anything that creates slow, regular waves in breathing, voice, movement, or balance tends to stimulate the vagus nerve and improve heart rate variability. Below is a list of rhythmic activities that have been shown to be effective. Keep in mind that if a client's unburdened system of parts has yearned to participate in any form of rhythmic activity not included on this list, encourage them to do so, as this list is based on research as of this writing and is not exhaustive.

1. **Slow paced breathing:** Inhale through the nose, using a count if that's helpful (inhale for a count of 4 and exhale for a count of 6), or simply relax, breathe in, and emphasize your exhale to be slightly longer. You can add a phrase or word on the exhale—like *calm*, *peace*, *relax*, or *ahh*—if desired.
2. **Humming and breathing:** Inhale quietly, then exhale with a sustained hum (often twice as long as the inhale). This practice is known as *bhramari pranayama*, or the "humming bee breath."
3. **Chanting:** Repeat a vocalization (e.g., *om*) at a comfortable pitch to naturally slow the breath and prolong the exhale.
4. **Singing:** Singing phrases and melodies (especially in choral or group formats) tends to naturally create slower, regular breathing cycles.
5. **Yoga:** Practice slow, repeated postures coordinated with regular inhale-exhale cycles, often found in sequences and relaxation practices (e.g., yoga nidra).
6. **Tai chi and qigong:** These are continuous, slow, repeated movement patterns, usually coordinated with diaphragmatic breathing.
7. **Dancing:** Engage in repetitive, rhythmic dance patterns at a moderate intensity.
8. **Rocking and gentle swinging:** Use low-frequency rocking or swinging (e.g., rocking chair, hammock) to stimulate the vestibular system.
9. **Rhythmic sound:** Listen to or create rhythmic sound or music that synchronizes with your heart rhythms (e.g., steady drumbeats patterned to your resting heart rate).

Seven Steps for Health and Balance of the Mind-Body

Tina, Ronan, and Leonie all reached a point in therapy when their protectors were ready to change their roles. Some changed all at once, like Tina's anxious, young protector who eagerly joined the unburdened exile on the playground. Other parts transition over time. After Tina unburdened the sad little girl who felt dread and emptiness, the fixer began to establish a more sustainable workload and the critic was becoming less extreme. Feeling less self-critical, Tina rekindled social connections and began participating in activities that she genuinely enjoyed, like Latin dance at the local performing arts center.

Once Ronan's Self helped his critical manager and rageful part understand their shame cycle, they identified their common motivation of keeping Ronan functioning despite the pain of the boy who had been bullied. The critic worried about the rageful part's effect on Ronan's reputation and self-respect, and while the rageful one understood this, it nevertheless continued its dedication to distracting with rage as soon as a whiff of shame emerged. After Ronan's Self helped the bullied boy transform his sense of worthlessness, Ronan showed up in Self-leadership to connect with other parts, like the suicidal part and the industrious hard worker. In doing so, he disrupted his shame cycle, and the rageful part began to notice more balance and felt ready for a change. In response, Ronan began to care for himself differently. His critic relaxed, he began to notice what it looked like to model balance, and he engaged in recreational activities like team sports, vacations with friends, and "just shooting the breeze" at the coffee shop. When he felt his stomach starting to churn, he listened. This change grew out of Ronan's awareness of "being unaware," which we will illustrate for you later in this chapter.

For Leonie, an obvious shift occurred when she realized that the self-sacrificing peacekeeper felt guilty for talking honestly with her therapist and was more interested in connecting with her mother than with her Self. This revealed the legacy burden of parentification, the dependency of her mother's exile on Leonie's caretaking part. Once her mother's exile's care was transferred to her own higher Self, things steadily changed. Leonie's peacekeeper could stop sacrificing her needs, and the angry part could be heard advocating for clear boundaries. Leonie also needed to retrieve the exiled girl from the trauma scene where she had felt helpless and ashamed for being unable to rescue her brother, Nick, from an assault by their father. At the same time, a part with homicidal thoughts emerged in its fantasy of saving Nick, which was a scenario clearly distinct from the dangerous, shameful character flaw that her parts had feared was lurking inside. These developments happened slowly, but Leonie's internal family system was still reaping the rewards as her health continued to improve.

Tina, Ronan, and Leonie came to therapy carrying shame from societal biases around race, gender, weight, individualism, ability, and scarcity—though in varying ways. While going into the past and rescuing their exiles had healed burdens of shamefulness, lasting integration came from cultivating present-moment awareness along with freeing their protectors from now obsolete roles. (See the following handout with *seven steps for health and balance* (Sowell, 2024), which provides a flexible blueprint for long-term systemic change and post-unburdening integration).

Seven Steps for Health and Balance of the Mind-Body

An IFS Path for Well-Being of the Internal System*

1. **Free yourself** from the past:** In conjunction with your Self and the Self-energy of trusted others (e.g., IFS therapists), continue to release underlying fears, shamefulness, or pain by returning to the unburdening steps.
2. **Develop ongoing awareness of stress in your internal system:** Keep the signs and symptoms of allostatic load (page 30) in mind so you can recognize the signs of a part in distress.
3. **When stressed, turn your attention inward:** Notice and reassure protectors who want you to turn away from distressed exiles. Your awareness of them is the first essential ingredient of unblending. Attend to sensations, feelings, thoughts, and urges. Parts notice you noticing them. Ask them what it's like to be noticed. Ask any exile who overwhelms you to try trusting you, at least a little, and dial down the extent to which they are sharing their feelings in the body. Then return to protectors to get permission to help the exile by going through the 6 F's.
4. **Open to compassionate connection with yourself and others:** This is your magic carpet. Notice the possibility for connection all around you.
5. **Listen for spiritual wisdom:** Invite your parts to be with you quietly. See what comes.
6. **Find or create relational support and community:** Find compatible, sustainable relationships. This can include the IFS community, a healthcare team with an IFS therapist, other health professionals, friends, and other communities of people on similar journeys.
7. **Move toward balance and wholeness:** Set priorities and cultivate daily practices and decisions by listening to your body for guidance as you attend to:
    - Food and eating
    - Sleep and rest
    - Work and leisure
    - Addictions and use of mind-altering substances
    - Physical activity and recovery time
    - Sustainable, satisfying relationships
    - Interests that feel good and right because they add beauty, meaning, joy, inspiration, and spiritual nourishment to your life

---

* Adapted from Sowell (2024).
** Note the difference between "your Self" and "yourself."

Achieving balance and sustainability in our lives requires honesty and the willingness to change. Are we expending energy in a way that is in balance with the energy being restored? Are we nourishing our bodies with the right nutrients? Does our physical activity keep us strong and flexible—and provide enough recovery time? Are our relationships in balance—with energy and resources flowing with mutual give and take in our relationships? True balance doesn't require perfection or equality; rather, it comes when both our needs and our resources are sufficiently sustained. Do the intellectual, emotional, and spiritual challenges we face stimulate growth, curiosity, and development, or do they overwhelm and leave us feeling depleted? By fostering this balance, we can support lasting health and well-being in a way that honors both our needs and our capacity to grow.

Relating to the Body

Once clients integrate unburdening, internal relationships soften, including with the body. While Tina, Ronan, and Leonie all arrived having burdened relationships with their body, changes were afoot for each of them.

Leonie

Leonie's social life was transformed ever since she began to set more sustainable boundaries with her parents. Her parts trusted and felt safe with her Self in the lead. She made progress on almost all fronts, but still struggled to sustain interoception—the awareness of the body's sensory signals that alert us to what's happening and what's needed. Interoception requires open access to physical sensation, which some of her protectors still feared. Although Leonie was pleased with her progress, she had yet to address her relationship with her body, which was fraught with a conflict between two parts with opposing roles: an anxious worrier who became hypervigilant in response to pain, and another part who avoided connecting with the body altogether.

When she reviewed the list of interoceptive signals from chapter 5 (page 77), she remarked, "I've been seriously disconnected from what my body's been telling me. I relate to almost all of the descriptions on this list—my sleep habits, how I eat or don't eat, not noticing when I'm getting sick or getting cold or even when my bladder is full. As I look back, I think this has been going on for a long time, like much of my life. It just got worse with the Crohn's."

Leonie's realization opened the door to exploring how protective parts took over when she didn't feel safe in her life. They protected her from overwhelm, but now this was interfering with her ability to register bodily cues. Parts protect us by shutting down or overriding bodily signals, especially when dissociation or inhibition are necessary for safety. As exiled parts leave the past, the Self can begin to walk with them in the present. With time and increasing safety of Self in the body, protectors are more willing to allow awareness of sensations like hunger, fullness, fatigue, pain, the need to stretch or take a break, and other cues that support health. The following exercise is designed to strengthen this process, helping clients be aware of the body's internal sensory signals and respond to them.

Experiential Exercise: Finding Parts That Shut Down Sensory Signals

Whenever you're not living fully in your body, it may be because a protector is distancing you from your sensory experience to keep you safe. Their efforts can range from mild disconnection to extreme dissociation. You may also have parts who notice your interoceptive cues but override them due to another agenda. This exercise can help you identify parts that disconnect you from your body's sensations or override and ignore those signals. It can also help clarify what you can do to stay more connected and attuned to your body's needs.

What body sensations or signals would be most helpful for you to notice to support your health moving forward? Check all that apply.

- ❒ Hunger, fullness, thirst
- ❒ Feeling hot or cold
- ❒ Heart rate and strength
- ❒ Breathing patterns
- ❒ Pain or muscle tension
- ❒ Need to eliminate
- ❒ Early indicators of illness (e.g., aches, chills)
- ❒ Touch, pressure, tingling
- ❒ Changes in energy (e.g., fatigue, sleepiness)
- ❒ Emotional body cues (e.g., butterflies, agitation, tension)

Which sensation or signal is your priority right now?

____

____

____

Describe a moment when you ignored or took a long time to notice that sensation or signal from your body. What was happening, and what did you feel in that moment?

____

____

____

How would you prefer to handle the situation if you could notice that sensation and respond in a new way?

____

____

____

What has stopped you from responding that way, or from being aware of the sensation in the first place?

____

____

____

How do you know when you're out of touch with that sensation?

____

____

____

Once you're done responding, notice feelings, concerns, action urges, or competing agendas that came up in response to the idea of noticing sensory signals. These are clues that reveal the part who ignores or shuts down interoceptive signals. Set an intention to follow the 6 F steps and connect with this part. It is most likely to be a protector. Spend time with it. Learn what it fears could happen if you felt these signals and what would make it safe. If it leads you to an exile, ask permission to circle back to the unburdening steps. If the exile has already been unburdened, this protector will need some updating and reassurance.

Having worked through the questions in the previous exercise, Leonie decided to prioritize the part who feared pain and would disconnect her from her body. She wondered how she might respond to it differently.

Leonie: Whenever I think about a medication change or the fact that I haven't settled into a new routine, I notice the part that leaves my body. Really, anytime I have a negative thought about pain when I'm not in Self, I'm either anxious—obsessing over every little pang of pain related to the Crohn's—or shut down.

Therapist: If you could notice the feeling and respond in a new way, how would you prefer to handle the situation?

Leonie: Fear is the problem. The Crohn's symptoms have stabilized and even improved. In my life and with my family, I'm much calmer. I'd like to feel hopeful . . . Well, I *do* feel hopeful when my parts give me some room. But I want to be free of this fear of pain. I can imagine living life by taking it as it comes, but I'm not there yet. I'd have to trust my parts . . . or maybe I mean my parts would have to trust me. That I will handle pain in whatever way works best.

Therapist: That makes sense, Leonie. Let's check in. Does the part who fears pain notice you? Does it notice all the positive changes you mentioned? It might need an update on the Crohn's disease and the young parts who have unburdened.

By tracking the onset of Crohn's in the year before it was properly diagnosed, Leonie found the overwhelmed teenager whose fear had launched an anxious protector and another protector who disconnected her from her body. With their permission, Leonie could now help the 16-year-old unburden her fear of physical pain and her confusion over being a diagnostic puzzle. In that year, she lost confidence in both her body and the medical system while receiving little validation for her grief over all the social activities and normal life she was missing in school.

After being seen, understood, and supported, Leonie's teenager was ready to release her burdens. She stood with Leonie at the edge of a field and watched her fear, sadness, pain, and mistrust disperse into sunlight. Afterward, she felt an openhearted appreciation for the support and guidance she was receiving, inside and out, and invited calm, courage, and confidence to flow through her body.

Finally, Leonie asked the anxious and dissociative protectors if they were watching and what they needed now. Were they ready to move on from their roles? Not quite, they replied. Instead, they opted to release half their workload and see how it went.

Tina

Tina's critical part had been leading with body shaming when she first came to treatment, blaming the snacker for her compromised cardiac and metabolic health. Now, cultural burdens about women's bodies felt "totally unacceptable" to her. She understood that the views she had internalized didn't match her values and had kept her from loving her body, but being aware of shaming "shoulds" was not the same as being free of them.

We are surrounded by negative messages about our bodies, including their size, shape, color, gender, ability, age, and every other feature. Tina reflected, "The messages from the Dominican and American history of colonialism have harmed me as a Black Dominican American woman. Even if I don't believe them, they're in me, like implants I need to pluck out so I can love my body. On some days now, I do feel like I'm taking care of my blood sugar, blood pressure, and cholesterol out of love. That's progress."

With her therapist's support, Tina experimented with and practiced honoring her body as the sacred vessel it truly was—the home of her internal family and the embodiment of her Self and the entirety of her life experiences. With appreciation for all she and her body had been through, and in the presence of her Self and her parts, she honored the body that had carried it all. She opened her heart. She felt the power of her Self alongside her parts, her own story, and her cultural history as she reconnected with her body. She trusted her therapist, who was white, with the full range of her experiences, but her lifeline was the Dominican community, especially a small group of women who laughed, grieved, and celebrated their own unburdening rituals together.

Ronan

Ronan had a long history of driving himself to physical and mental exhaustion: "I don't think about taking a break when I'm tired. My body has been a means to an end." His need to feel like a good person had always trumped his ability to listen to his body. Not only did he overlook immediate physical signals like fatigue and hunger, but he ignored chronic headaches, back pain, stomach upset, and joint pain.

After his young boy unburdened, Ronan realized that a protector had also exiled his body. "This part of me learned to not listen to my body. It just couldn't allow all that pain. It would have been too much for the little guy." Ronan was finally able to give his body some compassion after noticing a spartan teenager who had used the body as a means to an end, trading self-care for admiration.

"I can't believe how much I've ignored! The chronic pain, the sports injuries, and a lifetime of being off-balance. It all comes from feeling not good enough. I had to prove my worth constantly. I had to be successful—pedal-to-the-metal in everything. Now I know that boy and understand why my parts were so hard on the body. But here it is [*gesturing downward*] still paying the price! I apologize every day, every time my knee creaks or my shoulder aches."

The teenager was not entirely comfortable with this new attitude toward the body. He liked the heroism of ignoring pain, he liked feeling strong and pushing limits, and he desperately wanted to avoid looking weak. In response, Ronan rolled up his metaphorical sleeves and invested time inside to become the loving grown-up this teenager had needed and still longed for. Simultaneously, he insisted on taking care of the body, and also took responsibility for creating a kinder relational culture and a more balanced work life for his employees.

When the teenager was finally ready to release the inherited burden of rigid masculinity, Ronan sensed the higher Self of his father and grandfather standing with him and the teenager on the bank of the river where he had been baptized as a child. Panting and covered in sweat, they dove into the water together, floated to the surface, and lay on their backs companionably looking up at the sky. They didn't need to talk. They just floated, cool and refreshed, until they felt complete. When Ronan opened his eyes, he was back in the therapy office with an arm around the teenager's shoulders, and they were feeling the body together.

U-Turns for More Balance

IFS health therapy worked well for Tina, Ronan, and Leonie. While some people have less dramatic outcomes, many experience an important level of relief. We all have parts striving to survive and thrive who love to be appreciated—and really appreciate not being blamed and shamed. The practice of turning inward to identify and connect with parts, the U-turn described in chapter 3, is the act of choosing to be curious and focused instead of reactive and deflecting, choosing to be responsible for and to all of our parts. In the U-turn, we embrace the body and the inner community and claim the power of Self-leadership.

The U-Turn Process for Moments of Emotional Intensity

We guide clients through a U-turn when there is a "critical mass" (Schwartz, 2001) of Self-energy available to help them *pause* the immediate urge to act:

1. Invite the client to notice urgency and pause.
2. Help them shift the focus from the provoking situation or person to their internal experience.
3. Ask them to notice the energy of the urgent part with curiosity and an open heart.
4. Encourage them to ask the urgent part about its thoughts, emotions, body sensations, and behavioral urges:
    - What does it tell or show the client?
    - What behavioral urges does it have?
    - What is it afraid will happen if it doesn't react?
5. Facilitate connection between the client and the part. Invite the part to notice the client's Self-energy (presence, curiosity, understanding) flowing to the part.
6. Ask the part to trust the client to handle the situation.

The U-turn is an unblending strategy in which the client turns their attention around and talks with activated parts. Although it's not complicated or hard to understand, parts who believe they know best, feel righteously justified, or are busy countering feelings of shamefulness may not cooperate. Remember, managers aim to prevent, control, or contain feared outcomes. They do this in various ways, including shaming internally and trying to control circumstances and other people externally. When they receive interoceptive signals as threats, they will fear being disempowered and won't like being noticed.

Similarly, reactive firefighters will take over if an exile surfaces without permission and rattles the nervous system. A blended firefighter may opt for self-soothing or some kind of distraction, including blaming others. Aiming to put out an emotional fire, they are allergic to any hint of interference. They will not be disempowered, and they will rebel energetically against efforts to control their behavior. In these circumstances, the U-turn takes willingness, awareness, and practice. An external source of Self-energy can be the key to persuading fearful protectors to try something new.

Leonie's U-Turn Learning Process

After unburdening, it's not unusual for clients to return describing how protectors took over again. This is an opportunity. Protectors need attention when they don't trust or comprehend the full import of an exile unburdening. We take concerned protectors to revisit the exile and see how it's doing, we help the exile if the burden came back for any reason, and we discuss the protectors' needs. Burdens can easily revive in situations that are reminiscent of (or actually reprise) traumatic circumstances, such as holidays with family. Leonie came to session processing one such experience and was ready to try a U-turn.

THERAPIST: What do you most need today?

LEONIE: I want you to listen and understand. Then, I need to decide how I want to handle this with my father.

THERAPIST: Okay.

LEONIE: I know I need to listen to my parts, but for now I just want to tell you the story.

THERAPIST: No problem! I'll listen. What happened?

LEONIE: I was at my parents' house for dinner after work before going home. When dinner was over, my mother and I cleared the dishes while my father went to his study. A little later, my father walked to the foyer with his coat. He put his hand on the doorknob, turned to me, and said, "I'm heading out. Stay here with your mother tonight. She needs you." And he walked out before I could respond.

THERAPIST: I see. No explanation, no discussion, and no chance to speak.

LEONIE: You got it. I'm left holding the bag! He didn't even tell my mother he was leaving.

THERAPIST: What came up?

LEONIE: I caught my breath and noticed my angry part. Good, right? But there's more! When my mother saw his car leave, she came into the foyer and asked, "Where's your father going?" I told her what he said. I needed to go home to finish something before work the next day, but I felt anxious telling her. When I did anyway, she just walked back into the kitchen and kept on cleaning. I stayed to help her and asked if she wanted to talk about what happened. She said no. That was it. I was there another forty-five minutes before going home.

THERAPIST: Ready to focus on that inside?

LEONIE: [*Closes her eyes and focuses internally.*] I can feel parts who reacted.

THERAPIST: How do you notice them?

LEONIE: My heart is beating faster and a little harder. And my gut is churning, especially when I think of my father saying, "Your mother needs you."

THERAPIST: Any feelings or thoughts?

LEONIE: I hear, *What she needs is respect from her husband!*

Therapist: Who says that?

Leonie: That's a comment from the angry part.

Therapist: What do you say?

Leonie: It's true. My mother *does* need respect. In the past, I always stepped in when my father stepped out. Now I feel the anger.

Therapist: Is the angry part aware of you?

Leonie: Yeah, something is happening. I just felt the truth of all this and my heart and gut relaxed! That's a clear connection. The angry part is glad I'm listening. We appreciate each other.

Therapist: How does that feel for everyone else?

Leonie: Surprisingly, it's okay. I've avoided feeling angry for so long, but it actually helps. As long as I listen, it doesn't take over. That's the part who made me leave. I *knew* I had to go home.

Therapist: Wow, Leonie. That's big.

Leonie: It likes hearing you say that. And I like the physical relief. I had this thought *I have to stay.* But the angry part jumped right in—*You can't sacrifice your health again!* I knew it was right. I felt compassion for my mother, but also for my parts.

Therapist: How do they respond when you say that?

Leonie: They're relieved.

As Leonie told her story and spoke for her parts, she also listened to them. This is the Self-leadership we aim for in IFS.

U-Turns in Service of the Relationship with the Body

The U-turn is an obvious good option when clients talk about relational conflict. In IFS health therapy, we also use the U-turn to be in relationship with the body. First, we invite the client to notice how internal conflict affects their body. For example, after Ronan's exiled boy and teenager unburdened, he noticed when he got irritated about minor obstacles or resisted help. His therapist asked the following questions to identify this prickly part and learn what it needed: more unburdening, updating, or support while transitioning to a new role?

Experiential Exercise: Questions for Parts Who Can't or Won't Make a U-Turn*

The following questions are for the exile who feels pulled back into old beliefs or protectors who get back to work in old roles even though an exile has unburdened. Read each question, attend inside and, when you're ready, write your responses.

Describe the relevant circumstance.

____

____

Go back to that situation. What's happening in your body? Notice shakiness, gut churning, muscle tightening, hot or cold sensations, raised or lowered heart rate, rate of breathing, pain, shutdown, the urge to move, and so on.

____

____

What were you thinking?

____

____

What did you feel?

____

____

What did you want to do or say?

____

____

What did you do or say?

____

____

* Modified from Herbine-Blank & Sweezy (2021).

Can you feel curious, concerned, or compassionate toward this part now? If so, let the part know.

What worried or scared the part in that situation?

____

____

What vulnerabilities do you notice as you go back to the situation?

____

____

What unmet needs might underlie this part's concerns and reactions?

____

____

If this part is inclined to act, will this action feel good and right in your mind-body afterward? Why or why not?

____

____

How would your part need or want your Self to handle that situation if it occurred again in the future?

____

____

In doing a U-turn Ronan identified a competent, conscientious protector who was still trying to do too much. This part was afraid of Ronan failing and feeling shameful, and it would easily grow irritated. It wasn't aware that the exiled boy had unburdened, so Ronan introduced them. The protector was relieved and agreed provisionally to step back from working so hard to prove Ronan's worth. Ronan asked the part to let him (1) limit the amount of work he took on, (2) be more selective about the job contracts he accepted, and (3) plan some fun adventures. The part agreed.

Ronan's U-turns during integration helped him talk to his protectors about their needs. Some protectors need more time to adjust to a new role, especially in challenging situations like Leonie's interaction with her parents. Others need to hear that it's okay to revert to an old role when necessary. Yet others need more time to decide what's next or to practice new behaviors in less stressful contexts. Finally, a protector holding on to its role can signal that an exile isn't finished unburdening.

Balance and Sustainability

Tina, Ronan, and Leonie each started IFS therapy wanting help with health problems. Throughout therapy, they addressed experiences of neglect and physical, emotional, and relational harm that produced deep-seated negative identity beliefs (*I am . . .* unworthy, bad, and so on).

Tina came to IFS health therapy to address lifestyle changes recommended by her doctor, but went on a transformative journey to find a new way of being with her body, her past, and her parts. She released the internalized burden of fat shame and developed a loving, compassionate relationship with her body. Surrounded by a supportive network of women of color, she came to embrace activities like dance, exercise, and a tradition of shared cooking. She learned to enjoy a vibrant diet rich in fruits, vegetables, proteins, and ancestral foods seasoned with a hefty dose of social connectedness. Along the way, she lost the hallmarks of metabolic syndrome. Finally, she tapered down to occasional IFS health therapy maintenance sessions.

Ronan—who entered therapy with headaches, gastrointestinal distress, high blood pressure, and sleep disturbance along with neck, shoulder, and low back pain—was manifesting the emotional and physical burdens of childhood trauma. Years of bullying and physical abuse had left him feeling chronically ashamed, afraid, and stressed. Over time in IFS health therapy, Ronan experienced compassion for the boy inside, and his protective parts relaxed. Once they were free of extreme roles and polarized conflicts, his pain diminished, his sleep improved, and he began to feel safer in his body. This inspired him to do better in social relationships. With the support of his psychotherapist, he saw a physical therapist and tried out various physical practices like restorative yoga, rhythmic breathing, and gentle stretching and strengthening. He discovered that his body could tell him when he needed to rest. After three years of therapy, Ronan's new routines supported both his physical health and his mental well-being.

Leonie is still in IFS health therapy and feels hopeful about the future. As she continues to unburden her parts and resolve internal conflicts, she feels less stressed, anxious, and shameful. Her Self has become the "non-anxious presence for her anxious parts," allowing her to engage in more social and physical activities, like low-impact aerobic dance and singing with a choir. She has also invested in her relationships with cousins and extended family, joining them in various family traditions. She sees her parents regularly while maintaining sustainable boundaries. Leonie and her brother, Nick, live close to each other, share a commitment to recovering from trauma, and have a loving, supportive relationship. She describes a sense of interoceptive safety in her body, which lets her interrupt the stress-symptom cycle that can exacerbate protector roles and gut reactivity (Ge et al., 2022). Overall, she feels more confident, experiences less stress reactivity, and feels less pain. "I'm still learning how to take care of myself, but isn't everybody?" she remarked recently. ▌

Conclusion

Before the startling revelations of epigenetic research, the ACE studies told us that relational experiences affect physical health. And long before Dr. Richard Schwartz developed IFS, the field of mental health was well aware that relational experiences affect the mind. As we've illustrated throughout this book, IFS health therapy encompasses mind *and* body, revealing how external relationships in the past affect internal relationships, which in turn can influence behavior and affect the body's biological processes directly. IFS shows how curiosity can untangle all this. Curiosity is a lifeline when we fear what's going on inside.

When parts stay connected with external others by disconnecting from each other internally, they make the costly but imperative trade of self-knowledge and power for self-protection and external stability. Although children survive (and can even thrive) in challenging environments by making this trade, costs that lead to illness accrue in both mind and body. Illness is alarming, and serious illness turns life upside down, demanding often unwanted adjustments. At this point, we have reason to fear that we are the worst of our behavior. We are the behaviors driven by our vulnerabilities. We are unlovable. We deserve the shaming we received, the accidents we endured, the illnesses we suffer. When our protective parts respond to physical malfunctions by collapsing in fear, dissociating, denying, getting angry, or soothing in ways that accrue more costs (like using substances), we are at risk of feeling ever more helpless and hopeless.

In our view, IFS is well-matched for these experiences. Curiosity challenges the shaming, guilting, and pathologizing characteristics of manager parts inside and out, while kindness and compassion usher in the courage we need to pay attention to physical as well as emotional pain. In IFS, we do not sign on to control shamelessly reactive protectors or squash the feelings of denigrated exiles; rather, we make it safe for those parts to talk. *What do they fear? What do they want? What did they miss? What do they need?* Let's give it to them now. When we listen to parts, they listen to us. It may feel counterintuitive, but it works. Our parts can tell us about the body and translate for the body when it needs to speak. The internal system has a wealth of information and guidance for clarifying pain of any kind.

The body is a system with multiple subsystems. According to IFS, the mind is also a system with multiple subsystems. When a system's members support each other with respectful attention, validation, and assistance, the system comes into balance. By accessing our Self, the natural leader of the internal system, we can calm stress reactivity, grieve losses, and support the natural rhythms of the mind-body. Our mental and physical systems have this innate capacity to achieve balance and heal. We've shown you how—now give it a try.

[APPENDIX A]

Glossary of IFS Health Therapy Terms

The 5 P's: The traits or qualities of an IFS therapist: patience, presence, playfulness, persistence, and perspective.

The 6 F's: The steps that therapists use to help clients differentiate protective parts from the Self: find, focus, feel toward, befriend, flesh out, and (assess) fears.

The 8 C's: The qualities of the Self: calm, curious, connected, courageous, creative, clear, confident, and compassionate.

Alexithymia: Difficulty or inability of experiencing, identifying, understanding, and expressing emotions.

Allostatic load: The cumulative wear and tear from frequent or chronic activation of physiological systems that respond to the stress of life.

Autonomic nervous system: The nervous system that is spread throughout the body and controls unconscious, automatic processes like circulation, heart rate, respiration, digestion, and the functioning of our organ systems.

Blended: One part dominates consciousness so that we feel, behave, and think according to this part's emotions, impulses, and beliefs. We see the world and other parts through its eyes, and we are not aware of the Self.

Burdened: When a part accepts identity insults and holds malign beliefs about its (or another part's) value, it is burdened. The burdens often seem literal.

Burdens: Painful or disturbing sensations, negative beliefs, and extreme, suck feelings—all of which dysregulate us physically and emotionally. Parts often experience burdens literally (for example, as a backpack of rocks, an oily coating on the skin, sludge in the gut, or an extra organ in the body).

Co-regulation: The process of moving out of extreme autonomic or emotional distress.

Differentiation: See *unblending*.

Direct access: When a protector will not unblend, the therapist speaks to the target part directly while the client listens. Both forms of direct access (implicit and explicit) are methods of communicating with parts in IFS. The other method is called *insight*—it is described later in this list.

Do-over: During witnessing, the client's exile takes the client's Self (with help from the therapist as needed) to any place where it feels stuck in the past. There, it instructs the client's Self to do or say what it needed someone to do or say at the time. The exile may need help in more than one situation. When it says this is complete and it is ready to leave the past, the client's Self brings it to the present or a place of its choosing. This emotionally corrective experience is also known as *rescripting*.

Dysregulation: Stress-induced disruption of homeostatic balance among interdependent physiological systems and the internal family system of parts.

Exiles: Vulnerable, wounded parts who are stuck with extreme negative feelings, negative beliefs about their worth and identity, and painful or frightening physical sensations.

Firefighters: Protector parts that react to distract from or soothe pain when managers' preventive efforts fail to contain exiles.

Going inside: Devoting attention to a part with an inward focus characterized by curiosity.

Homeostasis: The maintenance of a relatively stable equilibrium between the interdependent physiological systems and the internal family system.

IFS health therapy: The application of IFS treatment to physical illness and health problems.

Insight: Our Self is consciously aware of a part and is verbally, visually, aurally, intuitively, or kinesthetically in communication with it. Also known as *internal communication*.

Integration: After an exile unburdens, the Self (1) checks to be sure protectors are aware of the unburdening and updates any parts who were not watching; (2) facilitates rapprochement between parts who have been in conflict; (3) asks protectors if they are ready to retire from extreme roles, asserts their freedom, and inquires about their interests; and (4) reviews beneficial shifts due to the willingness of protectors to try new things and exiles to release their burdens.

Interoception: The process of sensing and interpreting signals from inside the body that interfaces with the physical feeling of emotion.

Interoceptive signals: A sensory message sent from inside the body to the brain that indicates physiological state (e.g., muscle tension, heart rate, dryness of the mouth).

Invitation: The invitation is a feature of the unburdening process, which comes at the end, after the burden has been released. The Self invites the exile to take in whatever it would value going forward. Exiles typically name what they've been missing, like play, fun, freedom, love, and so on.

Managers: Protective parts that keep us functioning and act preventively to avoid overwhelm by exiled pain.

Mind-body: The complex intertwining of body and mind.

Neuroception: Our subconscious, automatic neural perception of what is safe or dangerous in our environment, including relationships.

Parts: Subpersonalities who have individual feelings, perceptions, beliefs, behaviors, memories, priorities, roles, and motives. These include protectors (managers and firefighters) and exiles.

Polarization: When protectors disagree and get into conflict about how best to survive, they are in polarization with one another. As protective tactics accrue unwanted costs over time, polarizations escalate, and protectors become more extreme. Conversely, when we meet each side with appreciation and curiosity, polarized parts deescalate.

Post-unburdening: The period following an unburdening in which the exile and other parts deepen their connections with the Self and experiment with their new access to Self-energy.

Protectors: Parts who seek to protect us from the pain of exiles—see also *managers* and *firefighters*.

Regulation: The capacity to return the interdependent systems of the mind-body to emotional, behavioral, and physiological homeostasis and to an optimal range of functioning.

Rescripting: See *do-over*.

Self: The other kind of consciousness, different from parts and innate to everyone, that is characterized by curiosity, calm, clarity, connectedness, confidence, courage, creativity, compassion, and openhearted love qualities that transform the way parts feel about themselves and how they behave inside and out.

Self-care: Self-led actions and decisions to care for one's physical, mental, and spiritual health.

Self-energy: The Self's relational energy.

Self-led: Seeing the world through the eyes of the Self and acting accordingly.

Target part: Inquiry in a session that focuses on this part. The client chooses the target part. If another part interferes and won't stop, it becomes the target part until it is willing to allow contact with the former target part.

Trailheads: Signs of a part being stuck in an extreme role and in need of help.

Unblending: A part withdraws its dominance and control of the client's consciousness. Parts can unblend and disappear, but we aim for them to remain present and be with the Self. Also known as *differentiation*.

Unburdening: The process of an exile releasing its burdensome beliefs and moving out of frozen, extreme feeling states. The steps of unburdening are witnessing and unblending, do-over or rescripting, retrieval, the unburdening ritual, the invitation, and integration.

Unburdening ritual: If an exile hasn't already unburdened spontaneously, we suggest a ritual. The part may wish to let burdens go to one of the elements (light, earth, air, water, fire) as in the shamanic tradition, or it may choose another way.

U-turn: Turning one's attention inside to notice somatic manifestations, feelings, thoughts, and the behavior of parts.

Vagus nerve: The primary and longest nerve of the parasympathetic nervous system, responsible for counteracting the sympathetic effects of stress on the body's organs. It extends from the head and throat (including the tongue, ears, and vocal structures) through the chest (heart and lungs), and down into the abdomen (stomach, gut, and intestines). The vagus nerve relays sensory information between the brain and multiple organ systems, regulating the function of the ears, larynx, heart, lungs, gastrointestinal tract, and immune system, and plays a vital role in reducing stress and inflammation.

Witnessing: The exile shows, tells, or in some other way communicates its experience to the Self, which validates, understands the experience and challenges shaming beliefs so that the part feels supported, accepted, known, and loved.

[APPENDIX B]

Feelings and Needs Inventory

The Feelings and Needs Inventory is an open access document developed by the Center for Nonviolent Communication (CNVC). It is enormously helpful when grasping the words to verbalize feelings and needs is difficult. It can be shared directly with clients as a visual prompt. The original materials can be accessed at **www.cnvc.org**.

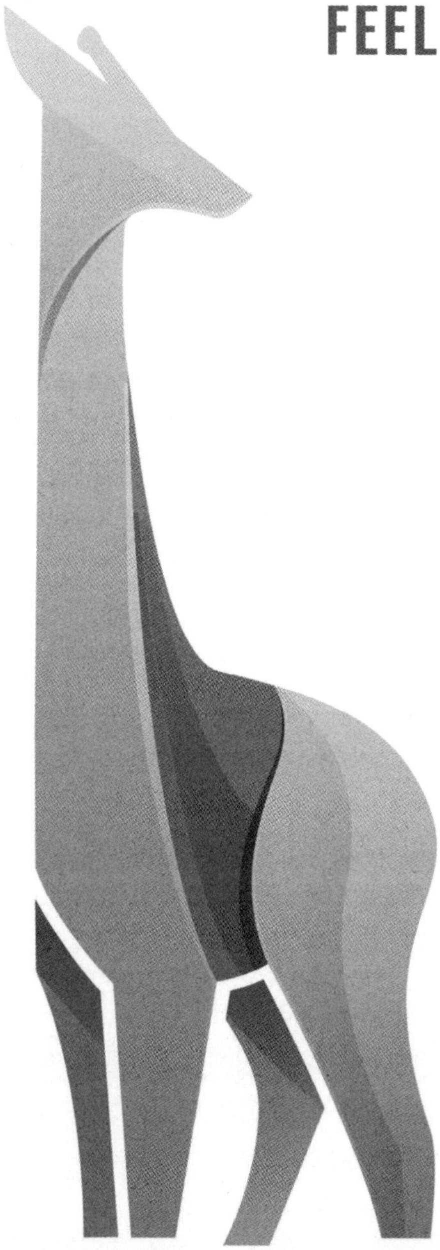

FEELINGS AND NEEDS INVENTORY

cnvc.org

The Center for NONVIOLENT COMMUNICATION

There are no positive or negative emotions, just emotions we feel when our needs are met and emotions we feel when our needs are not met.

— Marshall Rosenberg, Ph.D.

FEELINGS WHEN NEEDS ARE SATISFIED

AFFECTIONATE
compassionate
friendly
loving
open-hearted
sympathetic
tender
warm

ENGAGED
absorbed
alert
curious
engrossed
enchanted
entranced
fascinated
interested
intrigued
involved
spellbound
stimulated

HOPEFUL
expectant
encouraged
optimistic

CONFIDENT
empowered
open
proud
safe
secure

EXCITED
amazed
animated
ardent
aroused
astonished
dazzled
eager
energetic
enthusiastic
giddy
invigorated
lively
passionate
surprised
vibrant

GRATEFUL
appreciative
moved
thankful
touched

INSPIRED
amazed
awed
wonder

JOYFUL
amused
delighted
glad
happy
jubilant
pleased
tickled

EXHILARATED
blissful
ecstatic
elated
enthralled
exuberant
radiant
rapturous
thrilled

PEACEFUL
calm
clear-headed
comfortable
centered
content
equanimous
fulfilled
mellow
quiet
relaxed
relieved
satisfied
serene
still
tranquil
trusting

REFRESHED
enlivened
rejuvenated
renewed
rested
restored
revived

Increase your emotional vocabulary — are there more feeling words you can add?

The Center for NONVIOLENT COMMUNICATION
cnvc.org

2/4

FEELINGS WHEN NEEDS ARE NOT SATISFIED

AFRAID
apprehensive
dread
foreboding
frightened
mistrustful
panicked
petrified
scared
suspicious
terrified
wary
worried

ANNOYED
aggravated
dismayed
disgruntled
displeased
exasperated
frustrated
impatient
irritated
irked

ANGRY
enraged
furious
incensed
indignant
irate
livid
outraged
resentful

VULNERABLE
fragile
guarded
helpless
insecure
leery
reserved
sensitive
shaky

AVERSION
animosity
appalled
contempt
disgusted
dislike
hate
horrified
hostile
repulsed

CONFUSED
ambivalent
baffled
bewildered
dazed
hesitant
lost
mystified
perplexed
puzzled
torn

DISCONNECTED
alienated
aloof
apathetic
bored
cold
detached
distant
distracted
indifferent
numb
removed
uninterested
withdrawn

YEARNING
envious
jealous
longing
nostalgic
pining
wistful

DISQUIET
agitated
alarmed
discombobulated
disconcerted
disturbed
perturbed
rattled
restless
shocked
startled
surprised
troubled
turbulent
turmoil
uncomfortable
uneasy
unnerved
unsettled
upset

EMBARRASSED
ashamed
chagrined
flustered
guilty
mortified
self-conscious

FATIGUE
beat
burnt out
depleted
exhausted
lethargic
listless
sleepy
tired
weary
worn out

PAIN
agony
anguished
bereaved
devastated
grief
heartbroken
hurt
lonely
miserable
regretful
remorseful

SAD
depressed
dejected
despair
despondent
disappointed
discouraged
disheartened
forlorn
gloomy
heavy-hearted
hopeless
melancholy
unhappy
wretched

TENSE
anxious
cranky
distressed
distraught
edgy
fidgety
frazzled
irritable
jittery nervous
overwhelmed
restless
stressed out

cnvc.org
The Center for NONVIOLENT COMMUNICATION 3/4

NEEDS INVENTORY

PHYSICAL WELLBEING
air
food
movement/exercise
rest/sleep
sexual expression
safety
shelter
touch
water

HONESTY
authenticity
integrity
presence

CONNECTION
acceptance
affection
appreciation
belonging
cooperation
communication
closeness
community
companionship
compassion
consideration
consistency
empathy
inclusion
intimacy
love
mutuality
nurturing
respect/self-respect
safety
security
stability
support
to know and be known
to see and be seen
to understand and be understood
trust
warmth

PLAY
joy
humor

PEACE
beauty
communion
ease
equality
harmony
inspiration
order

AUTONOMY
choice
freedom
independence
space
spontaneity

MEANING
awareness
celebration of life challenge
clarity
competence
consciousness
contribution
creativity
discovery
efficacy
effectiveness
growth
hope
learning
mourning
participation
purpose
self-expression
stimulation
to matter
understanding

The feelings and needs presented here are neither exhaustive nor definitive. They are meant as a starting point to support anyone who wishes to engage in a process of deepening self-discovery, and to facilitate greater understanding and connection between people.

We hope you found it of benefit. Every day, around the world, CNVC aims to spread and support Nonviolent Communication so all may be inspired to become fluent in this *"Language of Life."* May you be inspired to pass it on. As a gift to you, and hopefully many others, you are free to share or copy this document; we request CNVC is credited as follows:

4/4

cnvc.org
The Center for NONVIOLENT COMMUNICATION

[APPENDIX C]

The Irreducible Needs of Children

The Irreducible Needs of Children, created by pediatrician Berry Brazelton and child psychiatrist Stanley Greenspan (2009), provides a clinically useful scaffold for identifying burdens of unmet developmental needs carried by exiled parts. Traumatic events are easier to recognize as sources of psychic injury than the daily erosion of self-worth that accompanies the absence of nurturance, attunement, and safe boundaries. We find it helpful to stay cognizant of these needs when talking with clients about burdens, communicating in direct access with parts, and identifying and finding burdened parts that may adversely affect health.

The Irreducible Needs of Children

1. **Ongoing nurturing relationships:** Nurturing relationships help a child to develop a well-regulated nervous system, enhance their flexibility and balance, protect them from over- and understimulation, and foster secure attachment.
2. **Physical protection, safety, and regulation:** Environmental and relational support and protection help children regulate emotionally and biologically.
3. **Experiences that are tailored to individual differences:** Respectful social interactions that recognize individual differences support brain, body, and identity development.
4. **Developmentally appropriate experiences:** Developmentally appropriate experiences with tolerable levels of challenge that include small positive outcomes build self-confidence, patience, and persistence.
5. **Limit setting, structure, and expectations:** Developmentally appropriate limit setting, structure, and expectations model reasonable boundaries in social relationships and respect for our own preferences and limits and those of others.
6. **Stable, supportive communities and cultural continuity:** Developing children need the positive regard of consistent, caring adults in schools and other social institutions to appreciate and support their cultural identity and heritage.

References

For your convenience, worksheets from this book are available for download at **www.pesipubs.com/IFSHealth**

Al Bekai, E., Beaini, C. E., Kalout, K., Safieddine, O., Semaan, S., Sahyoun, F., Ghadieh, H. E., Azar, S., Kanaan, A., & Harb, F. (2025). The hidden impact of gestational diabetes: Unveiling offspring complications and long-term effects. *Life, 15*(3), 440. https://doi.org/10.3390/life15030440

Bishop-Fitzpatrick, L., & Kind, A. J. H. (2017). A scoping review of health disparities in autism spectrum disorder. *Journal of Autism and Developmental Disorders, 47,* 3380–3391. https://doi.org/10.1007/s10803-017-3251-9

Boyce, W. T., Levitt, P., Martinez, F. D., McEwen, B. S., & Shonkoff, J. P. (2021). Genes, environments, and time: The biology of adversity and resilience. *Pediatrics, 147*(2), Article e20201651. https://doi.org/10.1542/peds.2020-1651

Brazelton, T. B., & Greenspan, S. I. (2009). *The irreducible needs of children: What every child must have to grow, learn, and flourish* (Rev. ed.). Grand Central Publishing.

Caglayan, S., Høye, A., Thimm, J. C., Wang, C. E. A., & Grønli, O. K. (2025). Association of adverse childhood experiences with physical illness and self-rated health in the population-based Tromsø Study. *European Journal of Public Health, 35*(3), 498–504. https://doi.org/10.1093/eurpub/ckaf031

Celano, C. M., Daunis, D. J., Lokko, H. N., Campbell, K. A., & Huffman, J. C. (2016). Anxiety disorders and cardiovascular disease. *Current Psychiatry Reports, 18,* 101. https://doi.org/10.1007/s11920-016-0739-5

Cené, C. W., Beckie, T. M., Sims, M., Suglia, S. F., Aggarwal, B., Moise, N., Jiménez, M. C., Gaye, B., McCullough, L. D.; American Heart Association Social Determinants of Health Committee of the Council on Epidemiology and Prevention and Council on Quality of Care and Outcomes Research; Prevention Science Committee of the Council on Epidemiology and Prevention and Council on Cardiovascular and Stroke Nursing; Council on Arteriosclerosis, Thrombosis and Vascular Biology; and Stroke Council. (2022). Effects of objective and perceived social isolation on cardiovascular and brain health: A scientific statement from the American Heart Association. *Journal of the American Heart Association, 11*(16), Article e026493. https://doi.org/10.1161/jaha.122.026493

Center for Nonviolent Communication. (2023). *Feelings and needs inventory.* https://www.cnvc.org/store/feelings-and-needs-inventory

Chakravarti, D., LaBella, K. A., & DePinho, R. A. (2021). Telomeres: history, health, and hallmarks of aging. *Cell, 184*(2), 306–322. https://doi.org/10.1016/j.cell.2020.12.028

Chapman, B. P., Fiscella, K., Kawachi, I., Duberstein, P., & Muennig, P. (2013). Emotion suppression and mortality risk over a 12-year follow-up. *Journal of Psychosomatic Research, 75*(4), 381–385. https://doi.org/10.1016/j.jpsychores.2013.07.014

Comeau, A., Smith, L. J., Smith, L., Soumerai Rea, H., Ward, M. C., Creedon, T. B., Sweezy, M., Rosenberg, L. G., & Schuman-Olivier, Z. (2024). Online group-based Internal Family Systems treatment for posttraumatic stress disorder: Feasibility and acceptability of the Program for Alleviating and Resolving Trauma and Stress (PARTS). *Psychological Trauma: Theory, Research, Practice, and Policy, 16*(Suppl. 3), S636–S640. https://doi.org/10.1037/tra0001688

Cree, R. A., Bitsko, R. H., Robinson, L. R., Holbrook, J. R., Danielson, M. L., Smith, C., Kaminski, J. W., Kenney, M. K., & Peacock, G. (2018). Health care, family, and community factors associated with mental, behavioral, and developmental disorders and poverty among children aged 2–8 years—United States, 2016. *Morbidity and Mortality Weekly Report, 67*(50), 1377–1383. https://doi.org/10.15585/mmwr.mm6750a1

Dariotis, J. K., Chen, F. R., Park, Y. R., Nowak, M. K., French, K. M., & Codamon, A. M. (2023). Parentification vulnerability, reactivity, resilience, and thriving: A mixed methods systematic literature review. *International Journal of Environmental Research and Public Health, 20*(13), Article 6197. https://doi.org/10.3390/ijerph20136197

Dolezal, L., & Bynum, W. (2024). Shame competence: addressing the effects of shame in health care. *Lancet, 404*(10462), 1514–1515. https://doi.org/10.1016/S0140-6736(24)02269-4

Felitti, V. J., Anda, R. F., Nordenberg, D., Williamson, D. F., Spitz, A. M., Edwards, V., Koss, M. P., & Marks, J. S. (1998). Relationship of childhood abuse and household dysfunction to many of the leading causes of death in adults: The Adverse Childhood Experiences (ACE) Study. *American Journal of Preventive Medicine, 14*(4), 245–258. https://doi.org/10.1016/S0749-3797(98)00017-8

Flores-Kanter, P. E., Moretti, L., & Medrano, L. A. (2021). A narrative review of emotion regulation process in stress and recovery phases. *Heliyon, 7*(6), Article e07218. https://doi.org/10.1016/j.heliyon.2021.e07218

Ge, L., Liu S., Li S., Yang J., Hu G., Xu C., Song W. (2022). Psychological stress in inflammatory bowel disease: Psychoneuroimmunological insights into bidirectional gut-brain communications. *Frontiers in Immunology, 13*, Article 1016578. https://doi.org/10.3389/fimmu.2022.1016578

Gescher, D. M., Kahl, K. G., Hillemacher, T., Frieling, H., Kuhn, J., & Frodl, T. (2018). Epigenetics in personality disorders: Today's insights. *Frontiers in Psychiatry, 9*, Article 579. https://doi.org/10.3389/fpsyt.2018.00579

Gold, S. M., Köhler-Forsberg, O., Moss-Morris, R., Mehnert, A., Miranda, J. J., Bullinger, M., Steptoe, A., Whooley, M. A., & Otte, C. (2020). Comorbid depression in medical diseases. *Nature Reviews Disease Primers, 6*, Article 69. https://doi.org/10.1038/s41572-020-0200-2

Herbine-Blank, T., & Sweezy, M. (2021). *Internal Family Systems couple therapy skills manual: Healing relationships with intimacy from the inside out.* PESI Publishing.

Herselman, M. F., Bailey, S., & Bobrovskaya, L. (2022). The effects of stress and diet on the "brain–gut" and "gut–brain" pathways in animal models of stress and depression. *International Journal of Molecular Sciences, 23*(4), Article 2013. https://doi.org/10.3390/ijms23042013

Holt-Lunstad, J. (2022). Social connection as a public health issue: The evidence and a systemic framework for prioritizing the "social" in social determinants of health. *Annual Review of Public Health, 43*, 193–213. https://doi.org/10.1146/annurev-publhealth-052020-110732

Hughes, O., & Hunter, R. (2022). Understanding the experiences of anger in the onset and progression of psoriasis: A thematic analysis. *Skin Health and Disease, 2*(4), Article ski2.111. https://doi.org/10.1002/ski2.111

Jemiyo, C., McGregor, B. A., Rehana, H., & Hur, J. (2025). Adverse childhood experiences and chronic health outcomes: Evidence from 33 US states in the Behavioral Risk Factor Surveillance System, 2019–2023. *BMC Public Health, 25*, Article 1650. https://doi.org/10.1186/s12889-025-22785-2

Kasarello, K., Cudnoch-Jedrzejewska, A., & Czarzasta, K. (2023). Communication of gut microbiota and brain via immune and neuroendocrine signaling. *Frontiers in Microbiology, 14*, Article 1118529. https://doi.org/10.3389/fmicb.2023.1118529

Larson, K., Russ, S. A., Kahn, R. S., Flores, G., Goodman, E., Cheng, T. L., & Halfon, N. (2017). Health disparities: A life course health development perspective and future research directions. In N. Halfon, C. B. Forrest, R. M. Lerner, & E. M. Faustman (Eds.), *Handbook of life course health development* (pp. 499–520). Springer. https://doi.org/10.1007/978-3-319-47143-3_20

Lin, J., & Epel, E. (2022). Stress and telomere shortening: Insights from cellular mechanisms. *Ageing Research Reviews, 73*, Article 101507. https://doi.org/10.1016/j.arr.2021.101507

Lin, L., Wang, H. H., Lu, C., Chen, W., & Guo, V. Y. (2021). Adverse childhood experiences and subsequent chronic diseases among middle-aged or older adults in China and associations with demographic and socioeconomic characteristics. *JAMA Network Open, 4*(10), Article e2130143. https://doi.org/10.1001/jamanetworkopen.2021.30143

Luo, X., Qiao, L., & Che, X. (2018). Self-compassion modulates heart rate variability and negative affect to experimentally induced stress. *Mindfulness, 9*(5), 1522–1528. https://doi.org/10.1007/s12671-018-0900-9

Mahmood, A., Simon, J., Cooper, J., Murphy, T., McCracken, C., Quiroz, J., Laranjo, L., Aung, N., Lee, A. M., Khanji, M. Y., Neubauer, S., Raisi-Estabragh, Z., Maurovich-Horvat, P., & Petersen, S. E. (2023). Neuroticism personality traits are linked to adverse cardiovascular phenotypes in the UK Biobank. *European Heart Journal–Cardiovascular Imaging, 24*(11), 1460–1467. https://doi.org/10.1093/ehjci/jead166

Maté, G. (2022). *The myth of normal: Trauma, illness, and healing in a toxic culture*. Avery.

Maude, H., Sanchez-Cabanillas, C., & Cebola, I. (2021). Epigenetics of hepatic insulin resistance. *Frontiers in Endocrinology, 12,* Article 681356. https://doi.org/10.3389/fendo.2021.681356

McCullough, L., Kuhn, N., Andrews, S., Kaplan, A., Wolf, J., & Hurley, C. L. (2003). *Treating affect phobia: A manual for short-term dynamic psychotherapy*. Guilford Press.

McEwen, B. S., & Akil, H. (2020). Revisiting the stress concept: Implications for affective disorders. *Journal of Neuroscience, 40*(1), 12–21. https://doi.org/10.1523/JNEUROSCI.0733-19.2019

Mikulincer, M., & Shaver, P. R. (2017). *Attachment in adulthood: Structure, dynamics, and change* (2nd ed.). Guilford Press.

Moriarity, D. P., & Slavich, G. M. (2023). The future is dynamic: A call for intensive longitudinal data in immunopsychiatry. *Brain, Behavior, and Immunity, 112,* 118–124. https://doi.org/10.1016/j.bbi.2023.06.002

National Scientific Council on the Developing Child (2014). *Excessive stress disrupts the architecture of the developing brain: Working Paper 3.* Center on the Developing Child, Harvard University. https://developingchild.harvard.edu/wp-content/uploads/2024/10/Stress_Disrupts_Architecture_Developing_Brain-1.pdf

Pietromonaco, P. R., & Beck, L. A. (2019). Adult attachment and physical health. *Current Opinion in Psychology, 25,* 115–120. https://doi.org/10.1016/j.copsyc.2018.04.004

Pietromonaco, P. R., & Collins, N. L. (2017). Interpersonal mechanisms linking close relationships to health. *American Psychologist, 72*(6), 531–542. https://doi.org/10.1037/amp0000129

Porges, S. W. (2022). Polyvagal theory: A science of safety. *Frontiers in Integrative Neuroscience, 16,* Article 871227. https://doi.org/10.3389/fnint.2022.871227

Porges, S. W., & Porges, S. (2023). *Our polyvagal world: How safety and trauma change us*. W. W. Norton & Company.

Rediger, J. (2021). *Cured: Strengthen your immune system and heal your life*. Flatiron Books.

Reyno, S. M., Simmons, M., & Kinley, J. (2020). A meta-analytic study examining the relationship between alexithymia and dissociation in psychiatric and non-clinical populations. *Research in Psychotherapy: Psychopathology, Process & Outcome, 23*(1), 26–39. https://doi.org/10.4081/ripppo.2020.439

Russell, M. A., Smith, T. W., & Smyth, J. M. (2016). Anger expression, momentary anger, and symptom severity in patients with chronic disease. *Annals of Behavioral Medicine, 50*(2), 259–271. https://doi.org/10.1007/s12160-015-9747-7

Satoh, H., Okazaki, K., Ohira, T., Sakai, A., Hosoya, M., Yasumura, S., Kawasaki, Y., Hashimoto, K., Ohtsuru, A., Takahashi, A., Watanabe, K., Shimabukuro, M., Kazama, J. J., Hashimoto, S., Kobashi, G., Ohira, H., Ohto, H., Kamiya, K. (2022). Relationship between risk of hyper-low-density lipoprotein cholesterolemia and evacuation after the Great East Japan Earthquake. *Journal of Epidemiology, 32*(6), 277–282. https://doi.org/10.2188/jea.JE20200267

Schwartz, R. C. (2001). *Introduction to the Internal Family Systems model.* Trailheads Publishing.

Schwartz, R. C., & Sweezy, M. (2020). *Internal Family Systems Therapy* (2nd ed.). Guilford Press.

Shadick, N. A., Sowell, N. F., Frits, M. L., Hoffman, S. M., Hartz, S. A., Booth, F. D., Sweezy, M., Rogers, P. R., Dubin, R. L., Atkinson, J. C., Friedman, A. L., Augusto, F., Iannaccone, C. K., Fossel, A. H., Quinn, G., Cui, J., Losina, E., & Schwartz, R. C. (2013). A randomized controlled trial of an Internal Family Systems-based psychotherapeutic intervention on outcomes in rheumatoid arthritis: A proof-of-concept study. *The Journal of Rheumatology, 40*(11), 1831–1841. https://doi.org/10.3899/jrheum.121465

Sharif-Nia, H., Jackson, A. C., Salehi, S., Miraghai, F., & Hosseini, S. H. (2025). Loneliness and repetitive negative thinking mediate the link between social health and cardiac distress in heart disease patients. *Scientific Reports, 15,* Article 11804. https://doi.org/10.1038/s41598-025-96968-7

Sharma, K., Akre, S., Chakole, S., & Wanjari, M. B. (2022). Stress-induced diabetes: A review. *Cureus, 14*(9), Article e29142. https://doi.org/10.7759/cureus.29142

Shonkoff, J. P., Slopen, N., & Williams, D. R. (2021). Early childhood adversity, toxic stress, and the impacts of racism on the foundations of health. *Annual Review of Public Health, 42*, 115–134. https://doi.org/10.1146/annurev-publhealth-090419-101940

Sonnenburg, J., & Sonnenburg, E. (2016). *The good gut: Taking control of your weight, your mood, and your long-term health.* Penguin.

Sonu, S., Post, S., & Feinglass, J. (2019). Adverse childhood experiences and the onset of chronic disease in young adulthood. *Preventive Medicine, 123*, 163–170. https://doi.org/10.1016/j.ypmed.2019.03.032

Souama, C., Lamers, F., Milaneschi, Y., Vinkers, C. H., Defina, S., Garvert, L., Stein, F., Woofenden, T., Brosch, K., Dannlowski, U., Galenkamp, H., de Graaf, R., Jaddoe, V. W. V., Lok, A., van Rijn, B. B., Völzke, H., Cecil, C. A. M., Felix, J. F., Grabe, H. J., Kircher, T., Lekadir, K., ten Have, M., Walton, E., & Penninx, B. W. J. H. (2023). Depression, cardiometabolic disease, and their co-occurrence after childhood maltreatment: An individual participant data meta-analysis including over 200,000 participants. *BMC Medicine, 21*, Article 93. https://doi.org/10.1186/s12916-023-02769-y

Sowell, N. F. (2020, May 20). *Questions for discerning the presence of a part.* IFS Health Therapy, www.ifshealththerapy.org

Sowell, N. F. (2024, August 16). *Seven steps for health and balance of the mind-body.* IFS Health Therapy, www.ifshealththerapy.org

Sroufe, L. A., & Waters, E. (1977). Attachment as an organizational construct. *Child Development, 48*(4), 1184–1199. https://doi.org/10.2307/1128475

Sun, Y., Li, L., Xie, R., Wang, B., Jiang, K., & Cao, H. (2019). Stress triggers flare of inflammatory bowel disease in children and adults. *Frontiers in Pediatrics, 7*, Article 432. https://doi.org/10.3389/fped.2019.00432

Sweezy, M. (2023). *Internal Family Systems Therapy for shame and guilt.* Guilford Press.

Taylor, K., & Demakakos, P. (2024). Adverse childhood experiences and trajectories of multimorbidity in individuals aged over 50: Evidence from the English Longitudinal Study of Ageing. *Child Abuse & Neglect, 149*, Article 106653. https://doi.org/10.1016/j.chiabu.2024.106653

Tong, R. L., Kahn, U. N., Grafe, L. A., Hitti, F. L., Fried, N. T., & Corbett, B. F. (2023). Stress circuitry: Mechanisms behind nervous and immune system communication that influence behavior. *Frontiers in Psychiatry, 14*, Article 1240783. https://doi.org/10.3389/fpsyt.2023.1240783

Turiano, N. A., Hill, P. L., Graham, E. K., & Mroczek, D. K. (2018, October 9). Associations between personality and health behaviors across the life span. In C. D. Ryff & R. F. Krueger (Eds.), *The Oxford handbook of integrative health science* (online ed.). Oxford Academic. https://doi.org/10.1093/oxfordhb/9780190676384.013.20

van der Kolk, B. (2014). *The body keeps the score: Brain, mind, and body in the healing of trauma.* Penguin Books.

Vineis, P., & Barouki, R. (2022). The exposome as the science of social-to-biological transitions. *Environment International, 165*, Article 107312. https://doi.org/10.1016/j.envint.2022.107312

Waldinger, R. (2015, December). *What makes a good life? Lessons from the longest study on happiness* [Video]. TED Conferences. https://www.ted.com/talks/robert_waldinger_what_makes_a_good_life_lessons_from_the_longest_study_on_happiness

Waldinger, R. J., & Schulz, M. (2023). *The good life: Lessons from the world's longest scientific study of happiness*. Simon & Schuster.

Weiss, A., Costa, P. T., Jr., Deary, I. J., Garside, D. B., & Stamler, J. (2020). The MMPI factor scales and risk of death in men during 45 years of follow-up: The Western Electric study. *Psychology and Aging, 35*(1), 97–111. https://doi.org/10.1037/pag0000421

Woo, E., Sansing, L. H., Arnsten, A. F. T., & Datta, D. (2021). Chronic stress weakens connectivity in the prefrontal cortex: Architectural and molecular changes. *Chronic Stress, 5.* https://doi.org/10.1177/24705470211029254

World Health Organization. (2023, March 7). *Disability and health.* https://www.who.int/news-room/fact-sheets/detail/disability-and-health

Xiang, A. H. (2023). Diabetes in pregnancy for mothers and offspring: Reflection on 30 years of clinical and translational research: The 2022 Norbert Freinkel Award Lecture. *Diabetes Care, 46*, 482–489. https://doi.org/10.2337/dci22-0055

Yaribeygi, H., Maleki, M., Butler, A. E., Jamialahmadi, T., & Sahebkar, A. (2022). Molecular mechanisms linking stress and insulin resistance. *EXCLI Journal, 21*, 317–334. https://doi.org/10.17179/excli2021-4382

Acknowledgments

Nancy Sowell

Writing a book requires stepping out of the ordinary flow of life, and for me the support of family, friends, and colleagues was essential. I'm profoundly grateful to my husband, Kim Comart, for his unwavering belief in my work, generously taking up the slack at home, and endlessly listening as this book unfolded. I thank my daughter, Melissa Febos, and daughter-in-law, Donika Kelly, always there to affirm that my experience was not uniquely flawed and offering the understanding and support of those living a writer's life. To my son, Barry Febos, for his understated wisdom, humorous relief, and playful vivifications with Angelo. I thank my Comart family—Jesse, Marissa, Ari, Lydia, and Liza—for the joyous interludes, ongoing interest, and sweet connections.

I thank my coauthors, who have been both friends and colleagues over many years of learning, coteaching, and collaboration, for their dedication to helping me write this book, going ever deeper into understanding the systemic impact of trauma and shame. Thank you, Martha, for encouraging me years ago to write a book, and for your steady support, clinical wisdom, and writing and editing virtuosity. I'm deeply grateful to you, Dick, for your trust, heartfelt support, and powerful, growth-filled learning and teaching experiences over many years.

I thank my early mentors in the IFS world who have taught me so much: Toni Herbine-Blank, Mike Elkin, Paul Ginter, Barb Cargill, Chris Burris, and Susan McConnell. I have deeply appreciated all of those who have taught beside me and influenced me as trainers and collaborators, including Jory Agate, Percy Ballard, Mona Barbera, Kathy Cox, Melissa Costa, Toni Crossen, Cathy Curtis, Fatimah Finney, Crystal Jones, Imma Lloret, Paul Neustadt, Larry Rosenberg, Joy Shivas, Sarah Stewart, Elizabeth Taeubert, Pilar de la Torre, and Deran Young.

I'm forever indebted to my clients, many of whom gave me permission to tell their stories, and all of whom have shared their inner worlds with me, helping me to become a more effective therapist for their internal system of parts. To my students, thank you for investing yourselves in the inherently vulnerable experience of learning something new.

I thank my friends for your loving, supportive presence, patiently listening to my thoughts and process: Toni Crossen, Cathy Curtis, Freddie Diamond, Jane Ginsberg, Ellen Karel, Mark Lange, Laura Lubin, Laura Roosevelt, Larry Rosenberg, Charlie Silberstein, Crickett Warner, Patricia Wild, Gerry Wright, and many more.

I thank Nancy Shadick and the research team in the Division of Rheumatology, Immunology, and Allergy at Brigham and Women's Hospital for the honor of cocreating the IFS rheumatoid arthritis intervention program in the first IFS randomized control trial. I thank the many IFS therapists who provided individual sessions in their private practices during that study, including Joan Atkinson, Fernando Augusto, Deborah Block, Fran Booth, Rina Dubin, Amy Friedman, Shelley Hartz, Suzanne Hoffman, Paul Neustadt, and Patricia Rogers. I'm deeply grateful to all the patients who enrolled in the study, trekked to the hospital for their IFS groups and sessions with me, and brought themselves so fully to the process.

Thank you to Zev Schuman-Olivier for your vision, support, and leadership, and for providing a home for IFS training at CHA. I'm grateful to you and the team at the Center for Mindfulness and Compassion for your investment in more IFS research on PTSD, intimate partner violence, and other applications.

Much appreciation goes to the IFS Institute leadership, including Jeanne Catanzaro, Katie Nelson, Donna Carter, Shawn Casselberry, and the entire IFS Institute team. Thank you to Jon Schwartz for the support and terrific teaching opportunities during your time at the Institute.

I am forever grateful for the international organizers Imma Lloret and Pilar de la Torre, Nicola Hollings, Vinciane van Outryve, David Schultz, Gus Murray and Elizabeth Keating, and the group at the IFS Association of France. Many thanks to all the international students and communities that have welcomed me, shared your culture and wisdom, and opened your hearts and homes in Ireland, France, Belgium, Sweden, and Spain. I'm grateful to the interpreters who have carefully translated my words and meaning: Cristina Pallí Monguilod, Helen Hernan, Anissa Vermeil de Conchard, Vinciane van Outryve, and David Convent. I thank the members of my advanced consultation group for their curiosity and connectedness—Imma Lloret, Norma Kisaiti, HeaKyung Kwon, Beth Rogerson, and Sandy Skezas.

I thank the many dedicated, talented people who have taught with me as program assistants through countless trainings, offering their time, expertise, and hearts. You have my deepest gratitude and respect. I wish it were possible to list every one of you here.

Writing a book on a subject that addresses the intersection of mind and body involves a wide field of influence from leaders in multiple disciplines. I have been fortunate to learn from many of them in person, while others have been my unknowing mentors. Some of these include Bessel van der Kolk, Daniel Brown, Ruth Lanius, Jon Kabat-Zinn, Lissa Rankin, Jeffrey Rediger, Stephen Porges, Deb Dana, Bruce McEwen, Nadine Burke Harris, Peter Levine, Laurence Heller, Alan Gordon, Gabor Maté, Robert Scaer, Sonya Renee Taylor, Allan Schore, Resmaa Menakem, W. Thomas Boyce, Michael Meaney, Rachel Yehuda, Dan Siegel, Howard Schubiner, Janice Kiecolt-Glaser, Herbert Benson, John Sarno, Antonio Damasio, Andrea Danese, Vincent Felitti, and Jack Shonkoff. Without your curiosity, explorations, and insight, this book would not be possible.

Finally, many thanks to the PESI Publishing team, including Linda Jackson, who helped me get started; Kate Sample, who saw this through to the end; and Jenessa Jackson, who provided the helpful combination of psychological sophistication and keen editing acumen.

Martha Sweezy

I'm grateful to Nancy for inviting me to participate in writing this important book and for her good-natured collaboration. I'm always grateful to Dick for being a brave visionary. And I thank Kayla Church and Kate Sample at PESI for their support of our process.

About the Authors

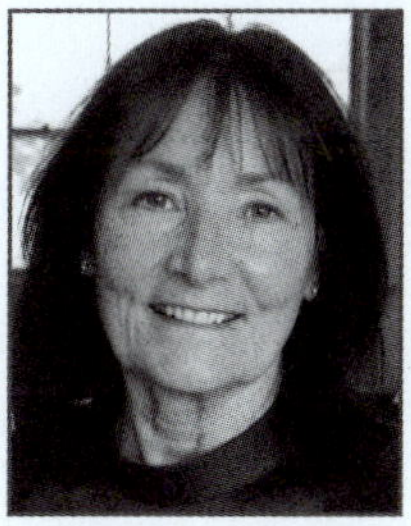

Nancy Sowell, LICSW, is an IFS senior trainer, consultant, and speaker who teaches internationally and in the US and maintains an IFS health therapy practice. She is a Harvard Medical School teaching associate at the Center for Mindfulness and Compassion at the Cambridge Health Alliance, where she has served for many years as a clinical consultant and IFS trainer. Her work integrates personal history, mindful awareness of the body, emotions, thoughts, and deeply held beliefs that influence our mood, behavior, relationships, and health. As the Behavioral Medicine program manager in the Division of Rheumatology, Immunology, and Allergy at Brigham and Women's Hospital in Boston, she co-created an IFS program that demonstrated positive outcomes for patients with rheumatoid arthritis. She knows both personally and professionally the power of the Self in healing and restoring health. Visit her website: http://www.nancysowell.com.

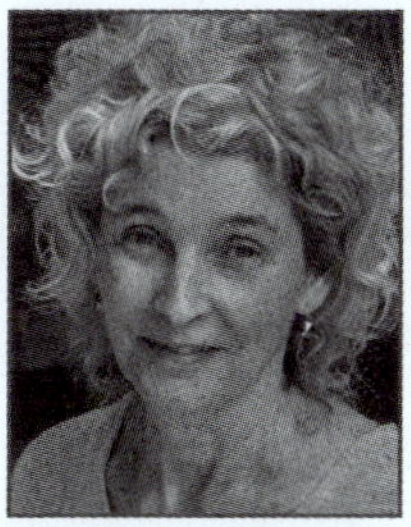

Martha Sweezy, PhD, is a part-time assistant professor in psychiatry at Harvard Medical School, a research and training consultant at the Center for Mindfulness and Compassion at the Cambridge Health Alliance, and a psychotherapist in private practice. She writes a blog on topics related to IFS in *Psychology Today* and cohosts a podcast with Hanna Soumerai-Rae and Fionna Kate Rice called *System Updates: IFS Chitchat*. She has authored, coauthored, and coedited ten other books on various applications of IFS, including *Internal Family Systems Therapy for Shame and Guilt*. She teaches IFS therapy nationally and internationally. Visit her website: https://marthasweezy.com.

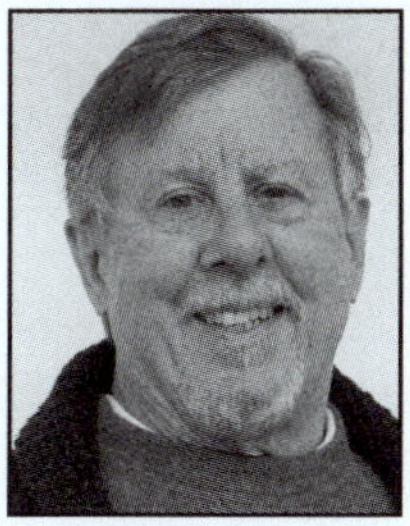

Richard C. Schwartz, PhD, is the creator of Internal Family Systems, a highly effective therapeutic model with a growing evidence base that depathologizes the multipart personality. Richard is also the founder of the IFS Institute, which primarily offers training for professionals. He is currently a teaching associate in psychiatry at Cambridge Health Alliance, a Harvard Medical School teaching affiliate. Richard has authored or coauthored more than ten books on Internal Family Systems and related topics, including *No Bad Parts* and *Internal Family Systems Therapy*. For more information on IFS, visit https://ifs-institute.com.